Ecaterina Mikitenko

The Book to Take with You for Childbirth

Publishing

The Book to Take with You for Childbirth

Ecaterina Mikitenko

Publishing
2022

This book is a true companion for women preparing for childbirth. It contains practical advice on breathing techniques, positions, and other self-help methods during contractions and pushing, as well as valuable information on postnatal recovery. You can confidently keep this guidebook with you as a cheat sheet that will be useful both during labor itself, and in the first days after childbirth.

TABLE OF CONTENTS

ABOUT THE BOOK

You are holding in your hands an amazing... No, that's not quite right. It is this book that holds you by the hand, leading you through sacred paths, paving the way through doubts, myths, and anxieties associated with childbirth. It will encourage, warm, and comfort you in a cozy blanket, enveloping you with the aroma of fragrant, aromatic tea and spices.

Can there be such feelings when considering childbirth and the postpartum period? Yes! This guidebook – this 'cheat sheet' – is written by Ecaterina Mikitenko, a careful, attentive, and deeply understanding doula. She has managed to create an atmosphere of the same care and delicacy in her book as she does in her work as a doula, combining this with her experience and knowledge, extending a supporting hand to all women preparing for childbirth.

"My dear!" – Katya addresses her reader, and immediately an intimate, confidential setting emerges and a conversation begins in which the story of childbirth becomes fascinating, filled with vivid images and subtle psychological observations. "... *Look at childbirth as a celebration... a mystery... a long-awaited day... of transformation... Childbirth is not just a medical event. It is also a deeply spiritual experience...*" writes Katya. I must confess, I read these pages with incredible pleasure, and when I reached the postpartum period, I realized that I would like to keep and use many of the recipes and much of the advice in my own practice!

This book is not just something to buy and read. It is one of those books that must be passed down for generations.

> *Svetlana Akimova is a practicing midwife, author, and facilitator of training programs for childbirth professionals and birth preparation courses, based in Moscow. She has been involved in this field since 1992 and is the founder of the Magic Baby Family Center (@magic_pregnant).*

There should be more books like this!

In the traditions of many cultures, there have often been protective talismans for birthing women that instill strength, provide protection, and fill them with warmth, accompanying them on their journey into motherhood.

I see this book as a unique talisman on one of the most important paths of a woman's life – motherhood! When reading this book, you can feel the author's presence in the gentle and wise guidance of birth and labor. Knowledge and human warmth, practical insights, and caring involvement – these are what every expectant mother needs on her journey towards becoming a mother, in her own unique and significant phase of life, including pregnancy, birth, and the early days of her baby's life.

This book will be of interest not only to mothers preparing for childbirth but also to fathers who choose to walk this path, supporting the women in their lives.

This book will also be valuable to those who accompany women during pregnancy and childbirth, as well as those interested in a holistic approach to perinatal psychology and psychosomatics.

I wish gentle and easy childbirth to the readers of this book and an exciting journey into parenthood, while

I wish Ecaterina a bright and exhilarating path in the field of perinatal support!

Gertruda Shpatakovska is a Doctor of Psychology (PhD), President of the Psychea Association, and Director of the Institute of Perinatal Psychology and Psychosomatics, based in Odessa. She is a family and perinatal psychotherapist (MIPU), a member of the Ukrainian Psychosomatic Association, and the All-Ukrainian Association of Art Therapy. Gertruda is certified as a body-oriented art therapist and a systemic constellation facilitator (France, Samadeva). Additionally, she is a trauma therapist trained in Eye Movement Desensitization and Reprocessing (EMDR, Austria).

PREFACE

Hello, my dear!

Giving birth is certainly not a time for reading, so it's best to read this during your pregnancy! However, this guide will be very useful to you during your childbirth, as a 'cheat sheet' where you can find important information, and as a talisman that will help remind you to believe in yourself and your own strength. So take it with you to the delivery room, just in case.

The idea to write this book came from women themselves who told me they took my previous book *Conscious Parenting* with them to the delivery room as moral support. However, *Conscious Parenting* is a collection of articles about preparing for conception, pregnancy, childbirth, and motherhood as a whole. So I decided to write a booklet specifically for childbirth: with practical advice on breathing, positions, and other self-help methods during contractions and pushing, along with valuable information about postpartum recovery. In short, I wanted to create a book that would become a real companion for women during childbirth and in the first days after.

This book is primarily aimed at women planning to give birth vaginally. However, if you have a planned cesarean section, you will still find a lot of valuable information in the second part of the book. Part one will also be beneficial for you, as even with a planned C-section, it is favorable to prepare for vaginal childbirth. This way, after the operation, you can have a sense of completion and the feeling that you gave birth, rather than it having been done for you.

If my book helps you during your childbirth experience, I would love for you to write to me about it. I would love to know that another woman has had a more joyful birth experience, and another baby has entered this world in a more harmonious way.

Please keep in mind that this book is purely informational. All the information presented in it is not medical advice, does not replace consultation with a doctor, and does not override the recommendations of a healthcare professional. The responsibility for making decisions and applying the information from this book rests solely with you.

I sincerely wish you a happy childbirth experience that you will remember with joy!

With love,
Your doula, Ecaterina Mikitenko

PART ONE

CHILDBIRTH

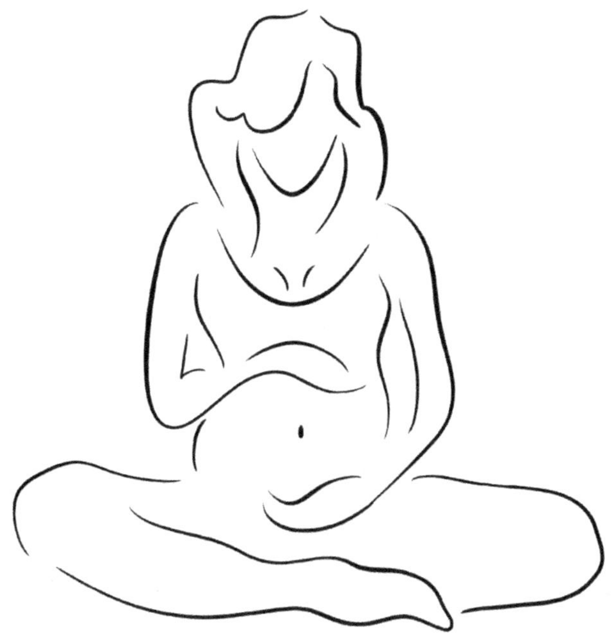

The day when childbirth begins is so exciting... especially if it's your first. On this day, you may experience many complex emotions: worry, anxiety, anticipation, and perhaps even fear. Do you know what I suggest? Look at childbirth not only as a responsible, challenging, and somewhat risky event, as people usually perceive it. Look at childbirth also as a celebration – the most important **celebration** for your family. Look at childbirth as a great **mystery** – the mystery of the emergence of a new human being into this world, with their own destiny and story. Look at childbirth as a **long-awaited day** – the day of meeting your child. And definitely look at childbirth as a **transformation** – your transformation, the birth of you as a mother.

Childbirth is not just a medical event. It is also a deeply spiritual experience. May you have a sublime and celebratory mood on the eve and day of your childbirth. This mood will help you overcome any negative emotions, any challenges, any pain, and any experience that you may encounter while giving birth to your child.

HOW TO TELL IF YOU'RE IN LABOR

Many mothers, especially first-time mothers, make the same mistake – they think they are in labor when it hasn't actually started yet! In other words, they mistake the early signs of labor for active labor. This leads to women expending physical and emotional energy when they could have been resting and conserving their strength for the upcoming challenging work.

So let's figure it out now: when do we consider that labor has definitely begun, and when do we realize that our body is still preparing for labor?

YOUR WATER HAS BROKEN

If your due date is approaching and your water has broken, that's great news. It's a sign that labor is very close. However, the rupture of membranes itself (also known as water breaking) does not necessarily mean that labor has started. From the moment your water breaks until the onset of contractions can take minutes, hour, or even days.

Each country has its own protocols here. In many countries, medical protocols allow for a waiting period of 24 hours for contractions to begin after the water breaks, as long as the mother and baby are in good condition. During this time, there is often no need to induce labor because the body needs time to initiate the process after the release of the amniotic fluid. Interestingly, in the United Kingdom, the protocol allows for a waiting period of up to 48 hours after the water breaks before intervention. According to some scientific studies, it is considered safe to wait up to 72 hours from the time the water breaks until the onset of contractions. It would be great if you could find out in advance what protocols regarding the rupture of membranes are followed in your country so that you know how much time you have. The good news is that in the overwhelming majority of cases, contractions start within 24 hours after the rupture of membranes. But as you already know, it's not necessary for labor to begin immediately after your water breaks.

Therefore, if your water has broken, it's important to note the time it happened, and pay attention to the amount of fluid, its color, and odor.

The color is very important! If the fluid is clear and transparent, that's a good sign. However, if it's green or has a foul smell, it means that the baby has passed meconium (baby's first stool) in the womb (normally, the baby only passes meconium after birth). This indicates that the baby may be lacking oxygen. In this case, it's important to seek immediate medical attention and be under the care of a doctor or midwife. Green fluid is not an absolute indication for a cesarean section, and the presence of green fluid doesn't necessarily mean that interventions will be performed, but monitoring the baby's condition by a specialist is necessary in such cases.

Regarding the amount of fluid, it can trickle slowly or gush out in a larger quantity, such as half a glass or a full glass. Don't worry: it's safe for the baby. Firstly, the baby still has over a liter of amniotic fluid inside. Secondly, the fluid is constantly replenished (every three hours), so babies rarely remain without fluid in the womb. Thirdly, the baby still breathes oxygen dissolved in the blood through the umbilical cord – not through the amniotic fluid, so if the water has broken, the baby won't start suffocating.

The real concern after the rupture of membranes is the potential for infection to enter the uterus through the birth canal. However, this almost never happens to healthy, examined women who follow simple guidelines. After the water breaks, it's important not to:

- Engage in sexual intercourse
- Bathe in bodies of water
- Insert fingers into the vagina (including frequent vaginal examinations).

These actions can introduce infection to the baby when the amniotic sac is no longer intact, so it's best to refrain from them.

Another important consideration is the position of the baby in the womb. If the baby is positioned transversely (horizontal), obliquely (diagonally), or breech (with the feet or buttocks down), there is a risk of the umbilical cord or the baby's leg prolapsing and protruding from the uterus into the vagina after the rupture of membranes. In such cases, it's important to be under the supervision of a midwife or doctor. However, if the baby is positioned head-down, the risk of cord prolapse after the rupture of membranes is almost nonexistent.

Thus, if the baby is in a head-down position and you eliminate the factors that could introduce infection into the uterus, after the rupture of membranes you can drink more water (to replenish the amniotic fluid), rest, go for walks, and rejoice that your meeting with your baby is very close. You can calmly wait at home for the onset of contractions for as many hours as allowed according to the protocol in your country.

If your water breaks at night, the best thing you can do is pay attention to the amount and color of the fluid and, if everything is good, lie down and rest. I understand that due to emotions and excitement, you may not be able to sleep, but try to at least lie down and doze off. The exact timing of when labor will begin, how long it will last, and when you will be able to sleep again is uncertain, so conserve your energy and rest! It is truly very important.

YOU HAVE STARTED HAVING CONTRACTIONS

If you have started having contractions, congratulations! It means that your labor has begun. The most important thing is to distinguish true contractions from false or Braxton Hicks contractions. Sometimes, even women who have given birth before find it difficult to differentiate between the two.

To help you discern better, remember that false contractions are irregular (the intervals between them constantly vary: sometimes every 10 minutes, then every half an hour, then every five minutes, and sometimes there may even be a lull). True contractions, on the other hand, are usually regular. They occur at consistent intervals for at least two hours (for example, every 15 minutes), or the interval between contractions gradually decreases over several hours (e.g., first every 12 minutes, then every 10 minutes, then every eight minutes, and so on).

How can you tell it's a contraction?

You will feel recurring, short-lasting (about 30-40 seconds) pulling pains in the lower abdomen or lower back (women often describe these sensations as 'cramping'). Yes, sometimes a woman may primarily feel the pain in her back, so keep that in mind.

If you have started having contractions, what should you do?

If you have a healthy pregnancy and no special risks, I suggest staying at home and monitoring how things progress, waiting for active contractions, which are strong and frequent. I adhere to the belief that it is safe for most healthy pregnant women to stay at home. Your home and its familiar environment can help you relax more easily. **Relaxation is one of the keys to having an easier and smoother labor.**

Moreover, while at home, you can engage in various activities to distract yourself from the pain. You can eat, take a nap, go outside to breathe fresh air, or spend some time in the shower – no one will tell you what to do or how to do it. And when labor enters the active stage (with contractions lasting about a minute and occurring approximately every three to five minutes for first-time births, or every five to seven minutes for subsequent births), you will have at least an hour to reach the maternity hospital without the risk of giving birth in the car.

Why am I in favor of waiting for active contractions at home if there are no concerning signs?

Firstly, childbirth is a natural and physiological process, meaning it is a healthy and normal process, and in the vast majority of cases, it is safe for both the mother and the baby if there is no medical intervention aimed at inducing, speeding up, or numbing labor without valid indications. In such cases, the risk of complications during childbirth increases.

Physiological, spontaneously initiated, and naturally progressing labors do not require constant monitoring and immediate hospitalization from the very first contraction. You might be surprised, but in the United States and some European countries, women may be denied hospitalization if their cervical dilation is less than four centimeters. Furthermore, in many developed countries around the world, some women even choose to give birth at home under the care of certified midwives (you might have heard about this), and it is legal and safe. Scientific research supports this approach.

I am not suggesting that you give birth at home if you have not specifically prepared for it. I am simply suggesting that you **spend as much time as is possible and comfortable for you at home**, ideally until active contractions begin.

The second argument in favor of experiencing the initial contractions at home is that childbirth, especially for first-time mothers, is often a lengthy process. You may find information online stating that first labors should last 9-11 hours, but natural childbirth can last 17, 20, or even 24 hours. Sometimes it can take even longer! However, in such cases, a doctor or midwife must monitor the baby's heartbeat and well-being.

Even in countries where home births are officially practiced, midwives transfer women to a hospital according to protocols if they have not given birth at home within 24 hours. This is at least the case in the Netherlands, which has the highest rate of home births in the world today.

So here's the thing: if a woman goes to the maternity ward with the first contractions, there's a high chance that she'll have to spend many long, tedious hours waiting for her labor to progress. This time can be spent more easily and comfortably at home. I will give you a list of ideas of what to do at home while you're waiting for the contractions to pick up a bit later.

Thirdly, it makes sense to stay home until active contractions because of hormones. Childbirth is a hormonal process, and the main hormone of labor is oxytocin – the hormone of love, and that's important to note. Oxytocin is a hormone that is produced in specific conditions, not in any situation.

The environment and atmosphere are crucial for oxytocin. It's a shy hormone that loves **darkness, silence, and warmth**. Did you know that labor often starts at night when it's dark and quiet? As you can imagine, it's not just a coincidence.

Oxytocin also loves the feeling of intimacy, safety, and relaxation. In bright light, noise, in the presence of strangers, in an unfamiliar place, when a woman is tense, this hormone is produced less effectively. Truly! It's the physiology of our bodies! And it's a fact that oxytocin will be better released in conditions where a woman feels safe, where she knows that no one will touch her or observe her, where she can draw the curtains, turn off the lights, enjoy silence, or play her favorite music.

This is not meant as a criticism of maternity wards. However, in most delivery rooms, the conditions are not exactly what oxytocin loves. Of course, there is an alternative: a synthetic analogue of our natural hormone of love. But... it's not as harmless as it may seem, and like any medication, it has side effects for both mother and baby. The question is: why create unnatural conditions for childbirth only to later treat them with artificial oxytocin? Wouldn't it be better to simply stay at home until the active labor phase?

Why do I often emphasize the phrase 'active contractions'?

Because the more active the contractions, the more oxytocin is produced, and **the more difficult it is to disrupt this delicate hormonal process**. Here's a rough example: when a train is just starting to move, it's easy to stop it, but when it's running at full speed, it's much harder to stop. The same applies to childbirth. Oxytocin is sensitive to the environment in which a woman finds herself – most especially during the early stages of labor. **Changing the environment in the initial phase of labor, unsuitable conditions for oxytocin production during early contractions – all of this can lead to prolonged, exhausting labor, weak labor activity, and even the cessation of contractions.**

I'll give you another example. The process of lovemaking is very similar to childbirth in terms of their hormonal cocktails – during sex and childbirth, the same hormones are produced. Is the environment important to you for intimacy? Would you be able to have sex in a hospital, in a brightly lit room, in front of other people, even if they were doctors? And even if you could, would you be able to relax and achieve orgasm? I'm confident that you wouldn't. You might argue that childbirth and sex are different things, but the hormones involved are the same, and we can't control hormones. They are produced in response to external factors and your emotions.

Of course, maternity centers are not established worldwide for no reason. They create a more comfortable, homelike environment for childbirth. There are special home-like rooms for giving birth in hospitals, where a woman can feel at home. If you think it's just a fad or someone's whim, my dear, believe me, it's not.

If you don't have the option to give birth in a home-like birthing room, then the most suitable environment can easily be created at home. And in the vast majority of cases, with a healthy full-term pregnancy and no special risks, it is safe to stay at home at least until the onset of active labor.

I'll reiterate: during the critically important period of hormonal adjustment and the 'rocking' of labor, being in the right environment is highly significant. It can even affect the course of labor overall by accelerating cervical dilation, easing childbirth pain, and avoiding unnecessary medical interventions. Of course, all of this is relevant if you have a healthy full-term pregnancy and can maintain relaxation and emotional calmness while staying at home until the contractions become very strong.

WHEN IS IT NOT POSSIBLE TO STAY AT HOME?

If you suddenly notice any of the following signs, it means that it is dangerous to stay at home, even if you had planned to stay home for longer. These are rare cases, but you should know that it is necessary to seek medical assistance urgently if:

1. There is bleeding: it is dripping, flowing in a stream, or blood clots are coming out. (Blood vessels in the mucus plug or the mucus plug itself being colored brown is normal.)

2. You feel a foreign body in the vagina.

3. There is a clear prolapse of the umbilical cord. This is a very dangerous situation, and you need to inform the doctors about it over the phone. Before arriving at the maternity ward, you should assume a position where your pelvis is higher than your head (such as the knee-elbow position) and find a way to keep the prolapsed umbilical cord moist (for example, by wrapping it with a wet towel).

4. There is pain between contractions. In normal circumstances, the pain ends with the contraction, and there should be no pain between contractions. Pain between contractions can be a sign of an incipient uterine rupture.

5. You have a severe headache and see spots before your eyes. This could be a sign of high blood pressure, which is dangerous during labor.

6. The amniotic fluid is green or greenish in color. (Transparent fluid is considered normal.)

WHEN TO GO TO THE MATERNITY HOSPITAL

This decision **is yours to make**. I suggested that if there are no risks, you can stay at home a little longer and go to the maternity hospital when contractions last about a minute and occur every three to five minutes for first-time labor. For subsequent labors, it would be earlier, around contractions every five to seven minutes, as labor can progress quite rapidly in subsequent pregnancies.

> **It is safe to stay at home for that long if you are within an hour's drive from the maternity hospital or birthing center, you have a healthy singleton pregnancy, and the baby is in a head-down position.**

However, if you feel anxious at home and you believe you'll only feel calm if you are in the hospital with a doctor or midwife from the onset of contractions, then it is your choice and your right. In that case, it makes sense for you to go to the maternity hospital immediately because **the most important thing in labor is for you to feel safe and able to relax**. Prioritize your comfort and well-being above all else.

You already know that oxytocin is the main hormone of childbirth. And you also know about the existence of the hormone adrenaline. When we are afraid or experience strong emotions, our body produces adrenaline in large quantities. And adrenaline has the ability to suppress the production of oxytocin. That's why when a female mammal in labor feels threatened, her labor stops so she can hide from danger and find a more suitable place for giving birth. The same applies to humans.

You should give birth where you feel safe. If you want to go to the maternity hospital with the first contraction or after your water breaks, then that is right for you. Just think about how you can create a 'warm-dark-quiet' environment for your labor in the hospital. It could be a dark eye mask, or polarized sunglasses that help darken the surroundings even in bright sunlight. You might also find headphones useful, playing pleasant and relaxing music to drown out any external noises. Or earplugs. You may also want to bring items that create a sense of comfort and remind you of home such as a blanket, decorative pillow, figurine, or a small painting. These familiar objects will help you alleviate the feeling of being in a hospital and make you feel that everything is okay and that you are safe.

By the way, even if you plan to spend most of the time during early contractions at home, these items can still be useful when you go to the maternity hospital. After all, the warm-dark- quiet environment and the feeling of safety are needed throughout the entire labor process, not just when contractions are starting.

WHAT TO DO AT HOME WHILE WAITING FOR ACTIVE CONTRACTIONS

The most important advice I can give you regarding childbirth is **to not focus on your labor for as long as possible**. Don't concentrate on your sensations, push away the thought that you're giving birth, and engage in some activity to distract yourself from contractions. Try not to notice your labor for as long as you can until the contractions become so intense that they bend you to the ground and you can't do anything else but get on all fours, crawl, or simply be on the floor.

I understand that this advice may sound strange and unfamiliar. It all relates to the physiology of childbirth. Labor is a function of ancient parts of the brain, alongside which we have a 'new' brain called the neocortex. The neocortex serves us well in everyday life as it enables us to speak, think, and invent things. However, during childbirth, the neocortex interferes because it inhibits the production of necessary hormones. The ability of the neocortex to suppress certain reflexive processes in the body is called neocortical inhibition, and it manifests acutely during labor.

External factors, especially light, noise, and speech, can provoke the activity of the neocortex, which, in turn, negatively affects the production of oxytocin. That's why the birthing environment is so important. However, we can also stimulate the neocortex ourselves through our thoughts, analysis, and control, thereby prolonging and complicating labor. Therefore, it is very helpful for the birthing process to distract ourselves from it. Focus on other tasks, and labor will progress naturally. Labor is essentially an uncontrollable process that simply occurs in our bodies according to a genetically programmed sequence. We just need to allow this process to happen without helping or hindering it!

If from the very beginning of contractions, we sit anxiously waiting for the labor to unfold, if we only think about it and agonize over it, constantly checking contractions on our phone, it won't lead to anything good! But if we engage in other activities, without waiting or constantly thinking about labor, that's when it will manifest itself much faster.

It is best, while contractions are still rare and mild, to come up with some kind of monotonous routine activity. It's a sort of meditation that effectively disconnects the neocortex and allows hormonal processes in the body to unfold as they should. You'll need to come up with a monotonous activity for yourself, preferably during pregnancy. I'll tell you a story for inspiration, shared with me by Gertruda Shpatakovska, and I found it quite delightful. It's a true story.

It happened in the summertime. A pregnant woman, not long before giving birth, decided to preserve tomatoes for the winter. She bought several kilograms of tomatoes, brought them home, and emptied them into the bathtub to wash them... and then she felt her first contraction. These weren't her first labor pains, and she knew it was the real deal. She realized that if she went to the maternity hospital now, gave birth, and returned home in two or three days, the tomatoes wouldn't wait for her. And she felt sorry for the tomatoes.

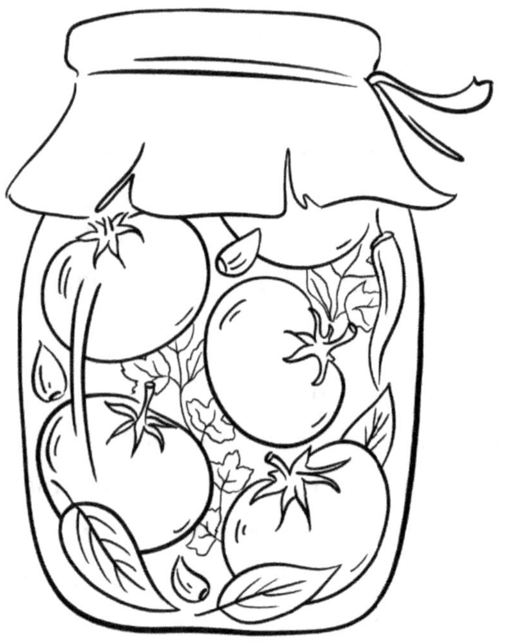

So, she decided to quickly jar a few bottles while she still had time. You can imagine the process of canning, can't you? It doesn't require much thinking, the actions are simple and repetitive, which allows the brain to disconnect and distract from the labor (plus, she had the motivation to finish canning the tomatoes before the baby's arrival). In the end, this heroic mother was almost on all fours when she sealed the last jar. Luckily, the maternity hospital was just across the road from her house, and she easily and quickly made her way there, where she gave birth shortly thereafter.

It would be great if you could come up with an activity like tomato canning to keep yourself from getting bored while waiting for strong, active contractions. Here are some ideas I have:

- **Check if you have packed everything in your hospital bag.** (Depending on the country of residence and the hospital, this list may vary).
  Here's a list of items for you and the baby:

  Items for you (for convenience, pack them separately from the baby's items)
    - Documents
    - Phone charger, phone, and headphones
    - Delivery gown (a beautiful new nightgown or robe – after all, it's a celebration!)
    - Extra change of clothes and a robe
    - Towel and toiletries
    - Washable slippers
    - Warm woolen socks (your feet may feel cold during and especially after labor)
    - Blanket (you might feel chilly during and after labor)

- Sleep mask or sunglasses (for darkness)
- Affirmation cards (more about them below)
- Rebozo scarf or a long shawl (for contractions and the postpartum period)
- Brewed tea or dried herbs for labor: a blend of mint, lemon balm, and oregano for contractions; and separately chamomile and chili pepper for prolonged labor (more about this below)
- Waterproof sheets
- Postpartum underwear or adult diapers
- Postpartum pads
- Wet wipes
- Paper towels or napkins
- Trash bags
- Water (at least 3 liters, you'll get thirsty during and after labor)
- Thermos with postpartum herbal tea for preventing excessive bleeding (details below)
- Thermos with a postpartum recovery drink (details below)
- Snacks (nuts, seeds, banana, chocolate bar, in case you get hungry during labor, and *chocolate actually stimulates contractions*)
- Honey (a spoonful of honey can give you strength if you get tired during labor)
- Drinking straw (it's impossible to drink lying down without a straw after giving birth)
- This book

- Postpartum first aid kit (chamomile, calendula, oak bark, nettle, yarrow, shepherd's purse, postpartum spices – more details in the second part of the book)
- Utensils (spoon, plate, cup)
- Essential oils and diffuser, if desired (more about them below).

Items for the baby
- Disposable or reusable diapers
- Disposable or reusable waterproof sheets
- Thin cloth diapers and burp cloths
- Several sets of clothes
- Multiple tops (onesies or shirts, as they often get soiled from milk and spit-up)
- Hat
- Blanket
- Cloth wipes or tissues (very convenient for wiping)
- Paper towels or napkins
- Wet wipes (let there be an extra pack in the baby's bag).

- **Prepare labor tea for yourself.** During labor, you can drink a tea made from equal parts of mint, lemon balm, and oregano. It's not mandatory, but this blend can help with cervical dilation.
- **Make postpartum drinks for yourself.** There are two types: healing tea for preventing excessive

postpartum bleeding (made from fenugreek or a mix of herbs like yarrow, nettle, and shepherd's purse) and a nourishing fruit and berry decoction for postpartum recovery. I'll provide you with all the recipes in the part two of the book, in *The first hours after Childbirth* and *Restorative beverage recipes.*

- **Cook yourself a restorative postpartum soup.** Postpartum nutrition is crucial, and I'll give you detailed information about it in the chapter *Your recovery*. It's great to have a hearty soup made from chicken broth in the first hours after your baby's birth. It will give you strength, energy, warm you from the inside, and nourish your body. You can prepare it while waiting for labor at home and take it to the birthing center or hospital in a thermos. This way, you'll have nourishing, restorative food right at hand after giving birth. It will be very helpful, trust me. I'll provide the recipe for this soup, which I learned from a Mexican midwife, in the second part of the book, in the chapter *What to eat for recovery*.

- **Bake a festive cake or cookie.** Birth is a celebration, and a celebration needs something special and sweet! Enjoy this dessert when the baby is born and truly celebrate his or her arrival in this world. Indeed, when I had my first son, I baked a cherry cake for his birthday. It was magical! And I've remembered it all this time.

- **Decorate the room.** Birth is your child's birthday and it's wonderful when the celebration is felt in all the details. To create a festive atmosphere, you can hang balloons, ribbons and flags. Just be careful not to climb too high though, you're in labor!

- **Go outside to a nearby park or your backyard.** Easy and safe movement stimulates contractions. Wear an absorbent pad or postpartum panty just in case your waters break or start leaking while you're walking. For a good mood, treat yourself to an ice cream or sweets during the walk.

- **Watch a movie.** Why not? Preferably a comedy. Laughing during contractions is beneficial – it can relax you a lot and contribute to a better course of the birth process. And you'll reduce waiting time.

- **Listen to your favorite music and dance.** Dancing is the best way to prepare the body for birth and the best way to gently stimulate contractions during the birth process. Plus, dancing improves your mood. And finally, today is a special day for you: you give birth to your long-awaited child!

WHAT HELPS DURING ACTIVE CONTRACTIONS?

While the contractions are short (30-40 seconds), infrequent (every 15, 10, 7, or even five minutes), and tolerably painful, try to distract yourself from the labor by focusing on something else. As I mentioned before, **try not to pay too much attention to the labor** while it's still possible.

However, if you start experiencing active contractions (every three to five minutes or more frequently) that are becoming difficult to ignore and endure, it's time to gradually start using various tools to cope with the pain. Your tasks during the active phase of labor are to:

1. Alleviate pain.

2. Relax as much as possible.

3. Disconnect your mind and surrender to the birthing process.

The ideas below can help you with these tasks during contractions. I'll explain each point in more detail:

- Breathing techniques

- Visualization and/or focused attention

- Sound or vocalization

- Positions

- Movement or dance

- Water

- Massage

- Essential oils

- Affirmations.

Not everything on the list may be useful to you. Some tools are universal (such as breathing, positions, and water), while others are highly individual. For example, one woman may require lower back massage from the first strong contraction until the pushing stage because it alleviates her pain significantly. On the other hand, touch may greatly irritate another woman. Some may find movement to be very helpful during labor, while others prefer to remain still and focus on their breathing. One woman may distract herself from the pain and disconnect her mind by making sounds, while another woman may prefer to remain quiet throughout labor and focus internally on the sensation of pain as beneficial or necessary pressure. All approaches are normal. By trying different techniques, you can choose from the list what works specifically for you. There is definitely something that will help you cope, make sure you discover it by practicing as much as possible before labor.

AND WHAT ABOUT EPIDURAL ANESTHESIA?

I'll put it this way: epidural anesthesia is **a medication**. A medication that was invented to treat pathological pain during childbirth in some women. And medication should be used when there are indications for it. Because like any medication, epidural anesthesia has side effects for both the mother and the baby. And in physiological childbirth, anesthesia is generally not necessary because we can manage labor pain without medication. Moreover, using anesthesia in physiological childbirth is an intervention in a natural process that is not justified because physiological pain does not need to be treated; it plays many important roles during contractions.

The pain in childbirth is not meant to punish women for the sins of Eve, who tasted the forbidden fruit in paradise. Pain ensures the physiological progression of the birthing process. If you want to give birth, then you need pain! Without it, labor can go awry. It is **thanks to pain** that:

- The cervix dilates (pain is involved in the hormone cascade, including oxytocin production).

- We naturally produce pain-relieving substances called endorphins during childbirth, which are essential for both us and the baby during labor.

- **We know how to move, breathe, and behave during childbirth because it is the pain that guides us, shaping our birthing behavior.**

- The birth of a baby becomes an even greater value to us.

- We form a bond with the baby being born (this has been confirmed in experiments on pain relief during childbirth in animals).

- Childbirth is safe (without pain, we would simply not realize that we are giving birth, and the baby could be born in an unfavorable place and under unfavorable circumstances).

- The process of producing breast milk is initiated (pain in childbirth stimulates the production of endorphins, which, in turn, promote the production of prolactin).

By removing pain from the complex hormonal chain of childbirth, we can disrupt the entire chain. This can lead to the need for various subsequent interventions, including a cesarean section.

Therefore, my dear, do not fear pain. It is your friend during childbirth, your helper. Embrace it. You just need to learn to collaborate with it. Let's focus on that now.

BREATHING TECHNIQUES

There isn't a single type of breathing that is considered 'correct' for childbirth. There are different techniques that work during labor – but remember the most important thing: **you need to breathe during contractions.** It is essential! Firstly, it actually helps alleviate the pain of labor. Secondly, it helps your baby receive an adequate amount of oxygen since they experience mild hypoxia during uterine contractions. Your oxygen supply is crucial for them.

I will share with you a breathing technique for contractions that I consider the simplest and most effective. It's called *Shh-Still*, and it was developed by Gertruda Shpatakovska. However, if you happen to forget about this technique during labor or if the *Shh-Still* breathing doesn't work for you, simply breathe in whatever way feels comfortable. **I'll let you in on a secret: since childbirth is an instinctive process, if you surrender to it, your body will naturally guide you on how to breathe, and that will be absolutely correct.**

So, let's try *Shh-Still* together. Take a calm, deep breath through your nose and exhale slowly and steadily through slightly parted lips. Release the air with a quiet sound. Pay attention to this sound – it resembles the sound of the ocean waves.

Try closing your eyes and envision this image: imagine yourself standing on the most beautiful beach, with gentle waves running up to the shore and receding back into the sea.

Keep breathing and focus on your breath and the sound of the 'ocean waves'. When you direct your attention to your breathing, you shift it away from the pain. Where your attention goes, energy flows. If you fixate on the pain during contractions, your sensations will intensify. But if you think about your breathing, making an effort to concentrate on the exhalation, making it very long and very slow, you relax and experience the pain more easily.

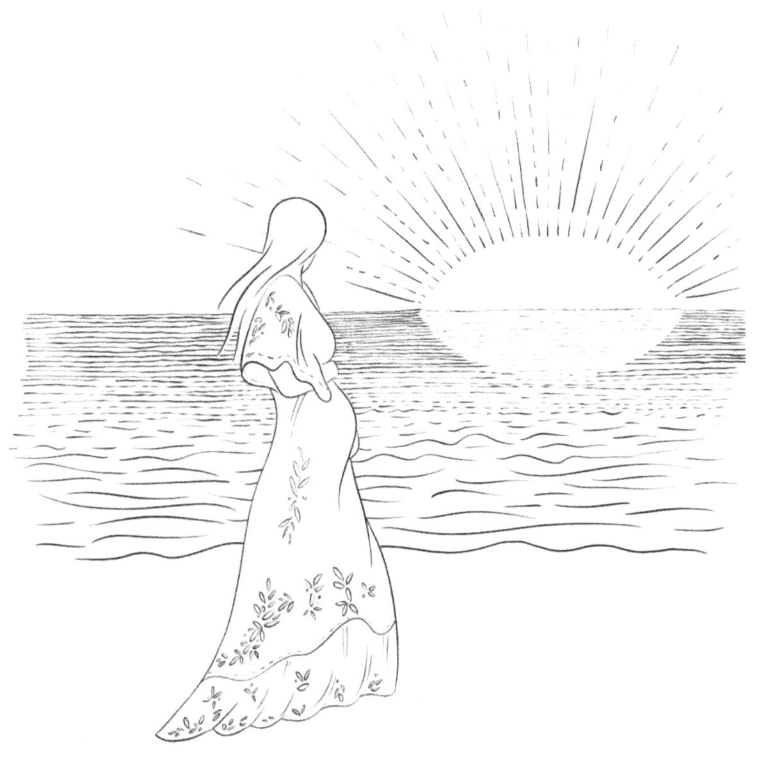

Adding visualization to your breathing will enhance the experience even further. Remember when you were imagining yourself standing on the seaside during your breaths? That's visualization. You can transport yourself to an imaginary place with each contraction. It will greatly distract you from the pain and help you relax more effectively. And **relaxation is the key to an easier and faster dilation of the cervix.**

I love visualizations for contractions. Imagine you're back on the beach – you see a small boat in the distance, and inside it is your baby, who will soon be born. Imagine with each contraction that the boat is coming closer to the shore. This movement cannot be fast because this vessel, carrying the most precious cargo, sails only with a gentle breeze. But each contraction brings the boat closer to land and your baby closer to you.

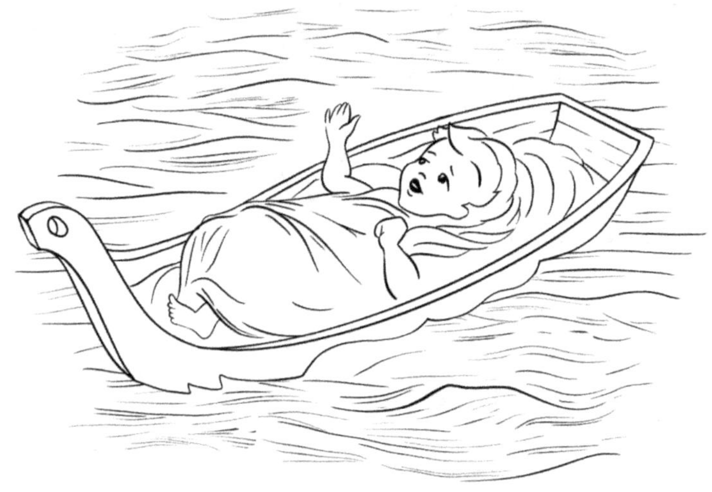

Alternatively, you can imagine a beautiful flower bud with a thousand petals. It could be a lotus or any other flower. Hidden at the center of this bud is your baby, and to see them, you must wait for all thousand petals to unfold and the bud to blossom. With each contraction, you can envision a new petal of your flower opening , **each new contraction undoubtedly bringing you closer to meeting your baby.**

You can come up with any image that comes to your mind for contractions. Remember to keep breathing throughout the entire contraction. If you don't feel like visualizing anything in your imagination, simply focus on your breathing and experience the contractions.

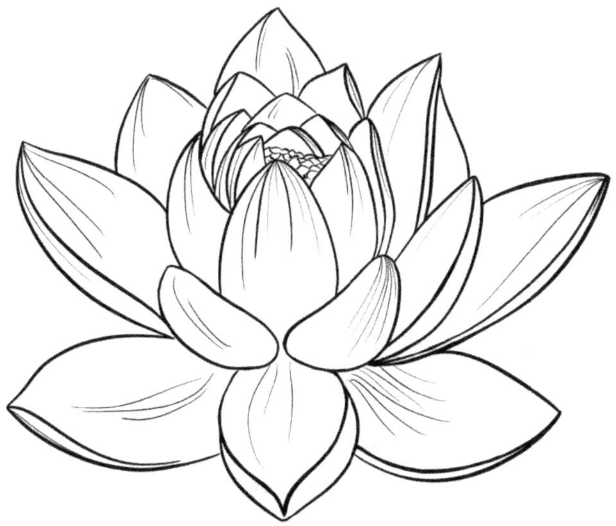

Focusing your attention on your baby can also be very helpful. When you think not about how painful and uncomfortable you feel, but about **how your baby is doing**, mentally communicate with them, explain what's happening, and encourage them, the contractions become much easier to endure.

Think about it: your baby is likely experiencing much more difficulty than you right now! Unlike you, they are unaware of why their previously gentle and loving womb has suddenly started squeezing and pushing them so forcefully, and they don't even know if it will ever end! Your support is crucial for them right now, dear.

When the contraction ends, relax and start breathing in your usual way. Find the most comfortable position where you can relax every part of your body to the fullest, and forget about everything: the pain you just experienced, whether the next contraction will come soon or not... Close your eyes, replenish your energy, and enjoy this break before the next wave and the next stage of work. **Use the time between contractions for rest – nothing else.** This is very important.

SOUND OR VOCALIZATION

When contractions become very intense and unbearable (approximately every one to two minutes), try using vocalization. You can still breathe using the "Shh" technique, but on the exhale, make a long and slow vowel sound like "a", "o", or "u". The "uuh" sound is particularly effective because it corresponds to the first chakra located in the pelvic area and cervix. Chanting the sound "u" on the exhale during each contraction will aid in the dilation process and distract you from the pain.

Please, don't worry about how it may appear to others. Childbirth is a process where **you have nothing to be embarrassed about**, especially if it helps you relax or cope better with your labor sensations.

POSITIONS

Just like with breathing, there is no right answer here. Each woman will find her own position for experiencing contractions, and, as with breathing, your body will guide you on which position is best. Sometimes women assume completely unexpected positions during contractions: standing on tiptoes, arching their lower back, or rocking while lying on a birthing ball. Some find it comfortable to stand during labor, while others prefer sitting on a birthing stool or toilet (by the way, many homebirth midwives like this position as it is convenient and effective), and some prefer to lie down for all their contractions.

Listen to your body and follow its lead! It knows better than anyone else which position will be most comfortable. Try different positions. Here are some common options that often work well for women in labor:

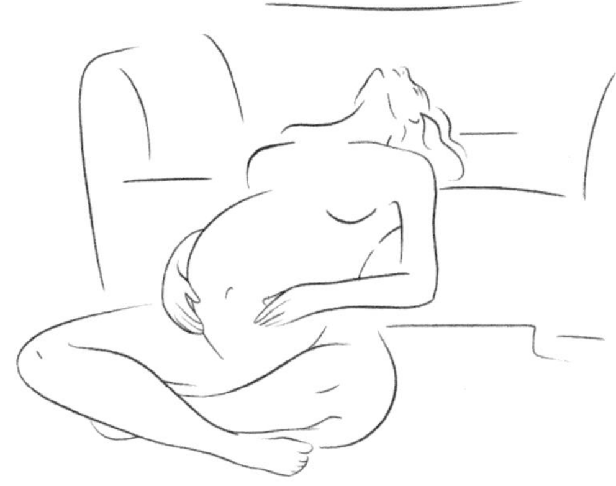

Sitting, hanging on the back of a chair or on the neck of a sitting partner.

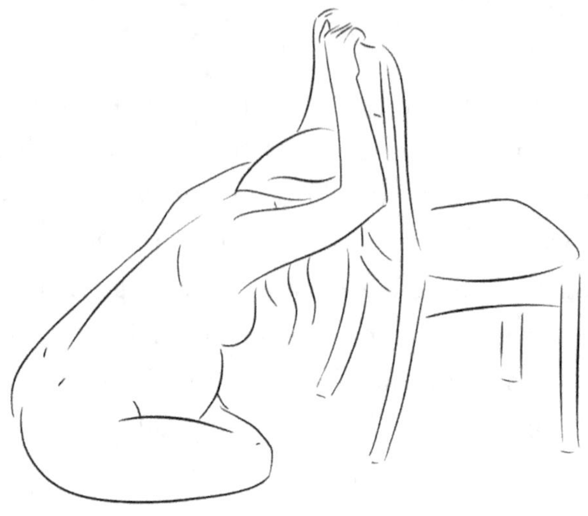

Sitting, hanging on the back of a chair or on the neck of a sitting partner.

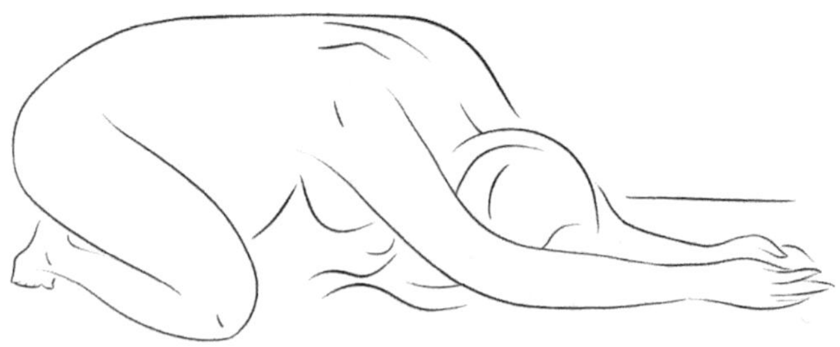

The 'sleeping baby' position ('child's pose' in yoga).

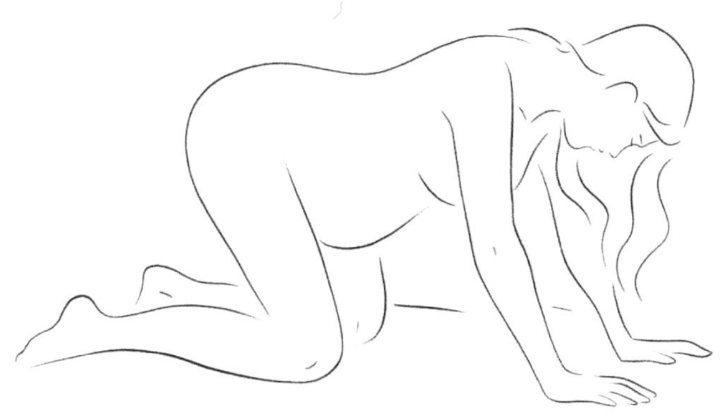

The 'cat' position

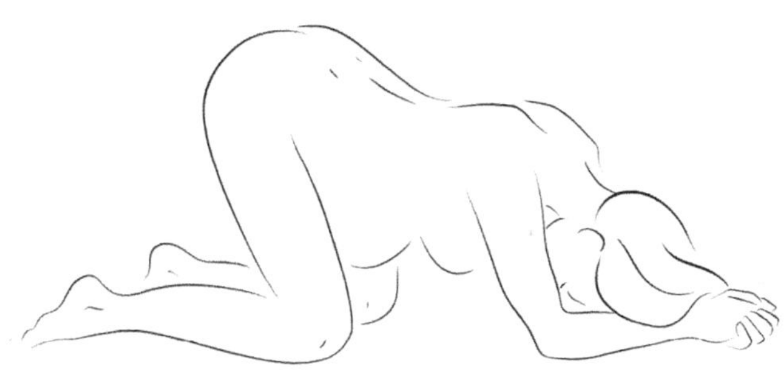

The 'cat' position with elbows on the floor

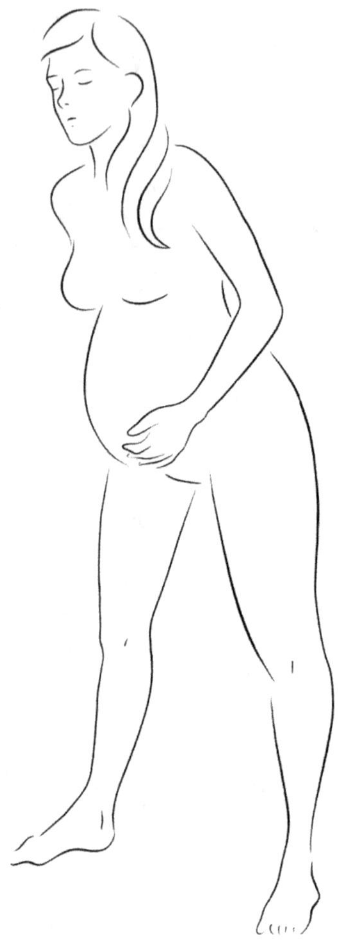

Standing, swaying hips.

Ecaterina Mikitenko

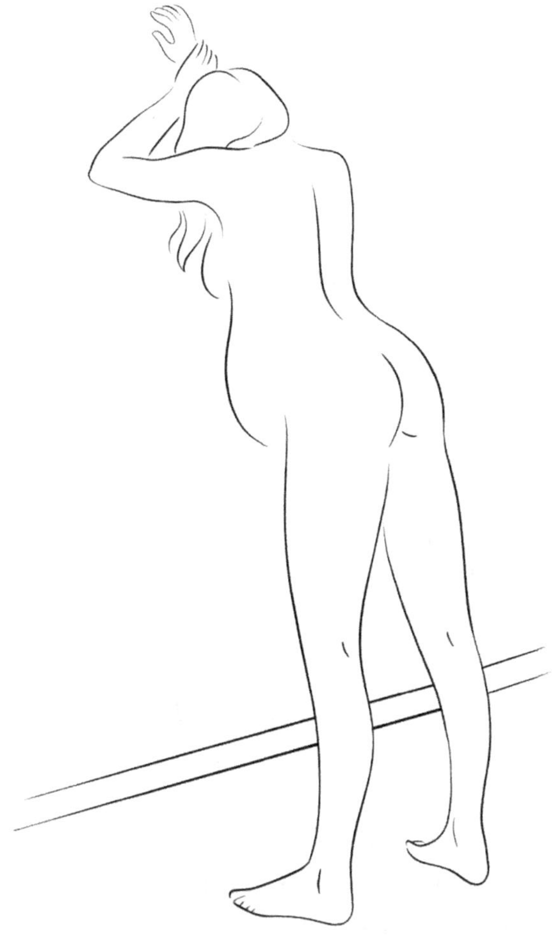

Standing, leaning against a wall, or hanging on the neck of a standing partner

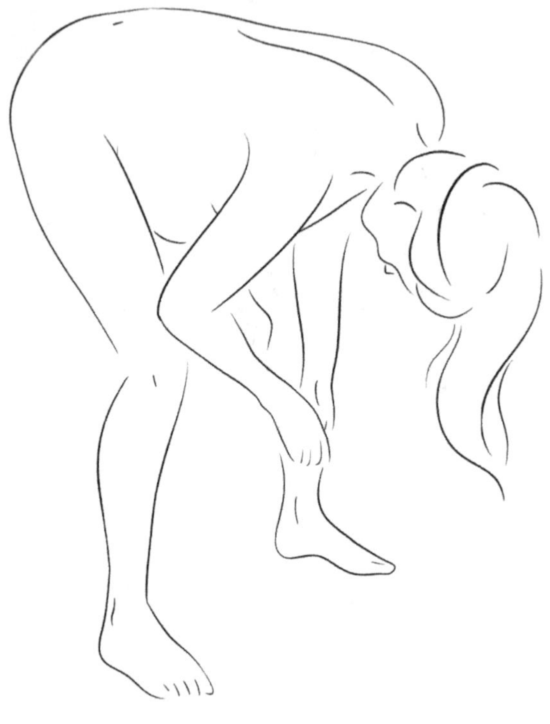

Standing, bending the knees and resting the hands on them.

No matter which position you choose, remember that towards the end of cervical dilation, especially if the labor has been long, it's important to conserve energy and **rest as much as possible between contractions**, so that you can recover at least a little during this short time after the overwhelming wave of pain. Therefore, during the active phase of labor when a contraction ends, please assume the most comfortable resting position where you can lower your head, lean on something, and relax every part of your body.

For example, if you were on all fours during a contraction, in the interval, rest your head and hands on the bed or chair, or sit on your buttocks and lean against the wall or chair, ensuring maximum comfort and avoiding staying in a position where your muscles might tense.

The resting position between contractions is just as important as the position during contractions. If you're comfortable in it and can relax, you can even doze off while your body prepares for the next wave. This is normal and even very favorable – to nap between contractions, especially if you're already very tired or haven't slept in a while.

MOVEMENT OR DANCE

You know what else helps many women during labor? Movement, especially hip circles and figure eights with the pelvis. Remember these two simple dance elements, they can become your allies during contractions or in between.

There is a whole approach to preparing for childbirth and behavior during labor called Dancing For Birth™. Its philosophy is that dance prepares women beautifully for childbirth and helps directly during the birthing process. I have trained in this method and practiced movements from our program with some moms during contractions. I can tell you that it really works!

You can rotate your hips or trace figure eights during contractions (if you feel like it). It will alleviate pain and promote better dilation.

WATER – BATHS OR POOLS

Water is perhaps the most effective way to reduce pain during contractions. It is a truly efficient, non-pharmacological pain relief method. Water relaxes the muscles, so the pain diminishes. So if you have the opportunity to lie in a bath or pool during strong contractions, it can be very helpful.

Just keep in mind some nuances about water during childbirth:

- It's best to immerse yourself in water when the contractions are already quite strong (being in water with minimal cervical dilation can slow down the already slow process of labor).

- Avoid staying in the water for too long – a few hours is sufficient (for the same reason: labor can become excessively prolonged).

- The water should be warm (when we're cold, adrenaline is produced, and as you already know, it's an antagonist to oxytocin).

If you don't have the option to lie in a bath during strong contractions, you may have access to a shower. Standing under warm water in the shower is also very effective during labor. Additionally, pouring water on the lower back with a showerhead or a bucket can alleviate pain. You can alternate between hot and cool water. Some women find such contrasting back rinses during contractions very enjoyable.

MASSAGE

The person who will be with you during labor should be the one to give you a massage: your partner, doula, mother, or sister. If you're in labor alone, you can try massaging your lower back or gently stroking your lower abdomen yourself, but it's not as convenient.

Here are some simple and effective massage techniques for the lower back:

- Circular kneading motions with the palms on the lower back.

- Rubbing the lower back with a figure-eight motion.

- Circular and linear kneading motions with the fingertips on the lower back.

- Gentle pressure on the lower back with fingers pressed together in a fist or the soft part of the palm's base.

You can also perform a gentle self-massage on the lower abdomen and inner thighs between contractions using soothing, stroking motions. Use a high-quality, therapeutic-grade lavender essential oil mixed with a carrier oil such as sesame, almond, olive, avocado, or jojoba oil. For every 5ml (1 teaspoon) of carrier oil, add 1 drop of lavender oil. You can prepare a bottle of this mixture during pregnancy for convenience.

ESSENTIAL OILS

Narrow-leaved lavender essential oil is a versatile oil that is suitable for almost everything. Importantly, it can be used during pregnancy and after childbirth. So, if you don't have a specific essential oil kit at home, preparing only lavender oil for labor will be a good choice.

In addition to lavender, other essential oils (also of therapeutic grade) can be helpful during labor: garden mint, peppermint, clove, jasmine, clary sage, geranium, frankincense, and orange. Each of them has different effects and methods of application. Some are suitable for warm and cold compresses, while others are used in diffusers or for indirect inhalation:

- **Lavender** calms, relaxes, and provides pain relief.
- **Garden mint** is also effective in relieving labor pain.

- **Jasmine**, **clove**, and **peppermint** stimulate uterine contractions.

- **Peppermint** also relieves nausea, reduces fatigue, and provides strength, especially during pushing.

- **Clary sage** and **geranium** calm and help with weak labor activity.

- **Frankincense** relieves psychological tension and induces a hypnotic state.

- **Orange** improves mood and invigorates.

Remember to choose high-quality, therapeutic-grade essential oils and follow the recommended dilution ratios and application methods. It's also a good idea to consult with a qualified aromatherapist or healthcare professional for personalized advice.

How to use essential oils

Attention: essential oils should be used in very small amounts! Essential oils should only be applied to the skin after dilution in a carrier oil (such as sesame, almond, olive, avocado, or jojoba oil). When adding essential oils to water, always use an emulsifier (cream) to prevent skin irritation.

Diffuser

When you feel tired and have accumulated a lot of psychological tension, try running a diffuser with 2-3 drops of frankincense essential oil for 15-20 minutes. It calms, dissolves negative emotions, and promotes relaxation. You can also rather use lavender, mint, orange, or any other scent that you find pleasant.

Inhalation from the bottle

If you don't have a diffuser, you can inhale essential oils directly from the bottle. Take a few deep breaths of the aroma of the oil that suits you best at the moment. This will be sufficient.

Indirect inhalation

Another alternative to a diffuser is to apply diluted essential oil to the skin. Dilute one of the oils mentioned above, depending on your needs, in a carrier oil (at a ratio of 1 drop of essential oil to 5ml of carrier oil) and rub it on your temples, the back of your neck, wrists, or under your nose. Alternatively, you can simply inhale the diluted oil from your palms.

Hip, sacrum, and lower abdomen massage

Dilute lavender or mint essential oil for pain reduction, or jasmine, clove, mint, sage, or geranium essential oil for stimulating uterine contractions in a carrier oil (1 drop of essential oil to 5ml of carrier oil). Gently massage the mixture onto your hips, sacrum, and lower abdomen. You can also massage your shoulders and back.

Warm compress on the sacrum

Apply diluted lavender, mint, jasmine, clove, or sage essential oil, depending on the situation (same recipe: 1 drop of essential oil to 5ml of carrier oil), and place a cloth (swaddling blanket or towel) soaked in hot water on top.

You can do it differently: mix a few drops of essential oil with a small amount of cream (this is the emulsifier for the essential oil, it must be used because essential oils do not dissolve in water). Add it to warm water (2-3 drops of essential oil per 300ml of water) and soak a cloth in it. Apply the cloth to the sacrum without prior oil massage. You can cover the compress with a dry cloth on top. The compress can be changed as it cools down. Thanks to the hot water, the essential oil will start to work faster, and the analgesic or stimulating effect will occur sooner.

Cold compress on the forehead

Put a few drops of essential oil (frankincense, lavender, peppermint, or orange) in a small amount of cream and add it to cold water (2-3 drops of essential oil per 500ml of water), soak a cloth in it, squeeze it and apply it to the forehead. This compress will help restore your energy if you're feeling tired. You can change the compress every five minutes as it warms up. You can also use cool aromatic water to wipe your face, neck, and hands.

Attention: if you haven't used essential oils before, please use them with caution during childbirth. Choose a maximum of two to three oils from the entire list and follow the rule: less is more. It is recommended to choose oils for childbirth one to four weeks before delivery when your body is already maximally prepared for childbirth, so that you can choose the essential oils whose scent will not irritate you during childbirth. The oils used must be ones you enjoy. Please do not exceed the doses and duration of oil application as indicated.

AFFIRMATIONS – THE POWER OF THOUGHT IN CHILDBIRTH

You know what else works great during childbirth? Affirmations – positive statements and short self-suggestions. It is our thoughts that give birth to our emotions and reactions (both physical and behavioral). What we think is important! It ultimately influences our behavior and our bodily sensations. Affirmations are great because they create a positive mindset, which is very important during childbirth. You can also use them during pregnancy. They are highly beneficial as they help alleviate anxiety, instill belief in your own strength, and help overcome various fears.

You can repeat affirmations silently in your mind, write them down on paper, or read them from cards. I suggest you prepare cards with positive affirmations in advance and put them in your labor bag, so that during the process of childbirth, you can look at them and support yourself. If you like, you can get creative with the design of the cards. Engaging in creative activities is so relaxing and fulfilling for a mother-to-be!

How to formulate positive beliefs? Avoid using the word 'not' and speak about something in the present moment.

Here are some examples of affirmations for childbirth. Many of them are taken from the Dancing For Birth™ program. You can use them or come up with your own! And if you hang cards with such phrases in your room during pregnancy, you will have more time for these positive programs to be created in your subconscious mind:

I am strong and calm.
I can handle any challenge.
I am filled with primal strength.
I trust my inner wisdom.
I believe in myself.
I trust in childbirth.
My body knows what to do.
My body knows how to give birth.
My cervix dilates easily during contractions.
My pelvis opens for my baby.

My perineal tissues are elastic and stretch well.
I easily release my baby into the world.

I want to share a story from my practice, which happened during the support of a mother's childbirth. It was her second birth, and they were progressing quite smoothly and quickly. The woman was already fully dilated, and contractions had begun, but the amniotic sac was still intact. This is completely normal and usually does not require intervention, but the midwife insisted on an amniotomy (rupturing the membranes).

The mother strongly desired for everything to be as natural as possible during her second birth and asked to wait for the sac to rupture on its own. The midwife agreed to give her an additional 10 minutes. During that time, the birthing woman began repeating aloud the phrase, *"My sac is rupturing on its own, and the waters are releasing"*. She repeated it over and over, calmly and confidently, fully focusing on her words.

The midwife glanced at her watch. By the end of the 10th minute, when time was almost up, the sac ruptured on its own! It was incredible! Since then, I have repeatedly used this example with other women to demonstrate the power of thoughts and belief.

During both of my pregnancies, I also worked with and wrote down various positive affirmations. I believe that this greatly helped me to approach my childbirth without fear, and to have the birthing experience that I had wanted. However, keep in mind that self-suggestions are not a magic pill, and there is no guarantee that all your affirmations will come true.

IF LABOR BECOMES PROLONGED

You have probably heard stories of someone's labor lasting for three days and the cervix dilating very slowly, or of someone experiencing frequent and intense contractions but no progress in dilation at all. In this chapter, I will tell you what you can do if you suddenly find yourself facing a prolonged labor, or if you are told that you have weak contractions.

Most often, in such cases, doctors suggest artificial oxytocin. However, you should know that this synthetic hormone has side effects and is not entirely safe. That's why its use should be completely justified.

For instance, the World Health Organization (WHO) does not recommend the use of oxytocin before the cervix is dilated to five centimeters if the mother and the baby are feeling well. Furthermore, the WHO believes that slow cervical dilation alone should not be an indication for oxytocin stimulation or the acceleration of childbirth.

In general, childbirth requires less stimulation than what is often provided. But even if stimulation is justified, my dear, know that there are many natural ways to accelerate the labor process, and you can try them.

The first and most important thing is your emotional state. How relaxed are you? How calm are you? If you're tense, fearful, or highly excited, the adrenaline that is produced during this time will hinder the release of oxytocin, and without oxytocin, labor cannot progress naturally! Try to relax using music, breathing techniques, or visualization, and eliminating factors that cause emotional or psychological tension. Try to let go of the situation and trust the process: allow labor to simply unfold with you. 'Surrender' to the process, release control, and 'dive' into your labor with all its sensations, without trying to resist, analyze, or understand them. This is the best thing you can do!

The second factor is the birthing environment. Remember how important the environment is during labor for the production of all the necessary hormones? Well, if labor is progressing slowly, check if all the necessary conditions for it are in place (warmth, darkness, quiet, safety, and intimacy). If not, try to create these conditions wherever you are. Turn off the lights, close the curtains, minimize external noises and sounds, refrain from talking to anyone, and immerse yourself. If it's cold, wrap yourself up or wear warm socks. Read more about what else you can do in the chapter *When to go to the maternity hospital.*

The third factor is rest. If you're feeling tired, if you want to sleep, it's understandable why labor isn't progressing –

your body is simply conserving its energy. You can sleep during labor! Trust me, you won't sleep through your labor. If you fall asleep, your contractions may completely stop for a while (especially if they were weak), and that's normal! Once you've rested and regained your strength, contractions will resume from where they left off. If you can't sleep, try to doze off and relax as much as possible. Just allow your body to take a break. When your body has had enough, the labor process will become more active.

The fourth factor is movement. The upright position is excellent for stimulating labor activity, as the force of gravity helps the baby's head press more firmly on the cervix and aids its dilation during contractions. If you feel strong and have the desire, you can take a walk (for example, in the park near the maternity hospital, or in your own yard) or sway or bounce on a birthing ball. Even better, play your favorite music and dance! Dance your baby into the world! Rotate your hips, trace figure eights. Active contractions won't keep you waiting for long.

The fifth factor is position. Sometimes the position a woman chooses to alleviate pain during contractions can slow the dilation of the cervix. In such cases, midwives advise changing positions and choosing those where the pain is felt more intensely. This is called "going into the pain", because the more intense the pain, the faster the cervix dilates. There is also a tactic called the "rule of three contractions". To determine which position is most effective for cervical dilation, midwives recommend staying in one position for three contractions and then switching to another. The position where progress is observed and felt is the one to stick with. The "toilet seat" position (which can be taken on a real toilet or a birthing stool) with legs spread wide apart and the torso slightly leaning forward is often very effective. Additionally, it is a vertical position, and gravity is our great friend during labor! This includes squatting and crawling on all fours.

The sixth factor is massaging oxytocin points. These are located on the hands between the thumbs and index fingers. During contractions or in between them, massage this point on one hand or the other, or rhythmically press on it. This will enhance uterine contractions.

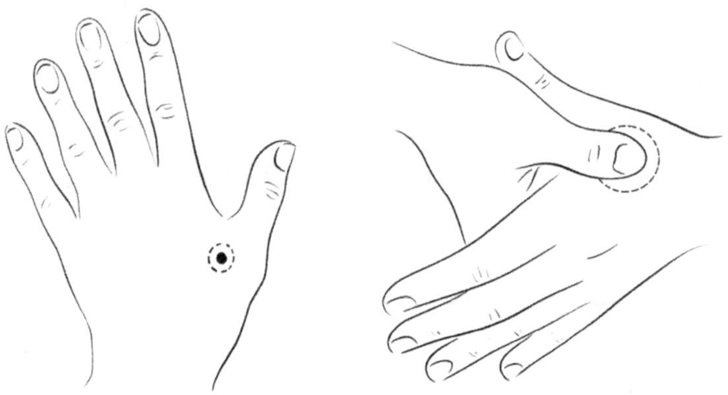

The seventh factor is kissing and caressing from your partner, gentle and arousing breast massage, and nipple stimulation in an intimate setting (without any onlookers!). Kisses and caresses can relax a woman

                                        Ecaterina Mikitenko

better than any medication (yes, during labor, can you imagine?). Kisses, among other things, relax your lips, and the mouth is a projection of the cervix. When the lips are relaxed during labor, cervical dilation becomes easier. And of course, kisses and caresses will contribute to the production of natural oxytocin, which is very beneficial. Some women, during labor, especially in the early stages, may even engage in intimate relations with their partner. Typically, this can significantly speed up and facilitate the process of cervical dilation.

The eighth factor is dark chocolate. Many midwives suggest having it on hand as a natural stimulator of the birthing process. Cocoa can be used instead.

The ninth factor is chamomile with chili pepper. Mexican midwives believe that the cause of weak contractions is a 'cold' uterus. An infusion of chamomile with chili pepper warms the uterus. According to the experience of midwives in Mexico, this drink works wonderfully where there is a need to strengthen uterine contractions.

The tenth factor is rebozo massage for the perineum. Take a rebozo scarf or simply a long shawl, wrap it around your hips in the perineal area as shown in the illustration, and ask your midwife, doula or partner to give you a massage by stretching the ends of the rebozo alternately. If you are alone during labor, place the center of the shawl between your hips in the perineal area and pull on the ends one by one, giving yourself a stimulating

self-massage of the perineum. This greatly enhances
contractions.

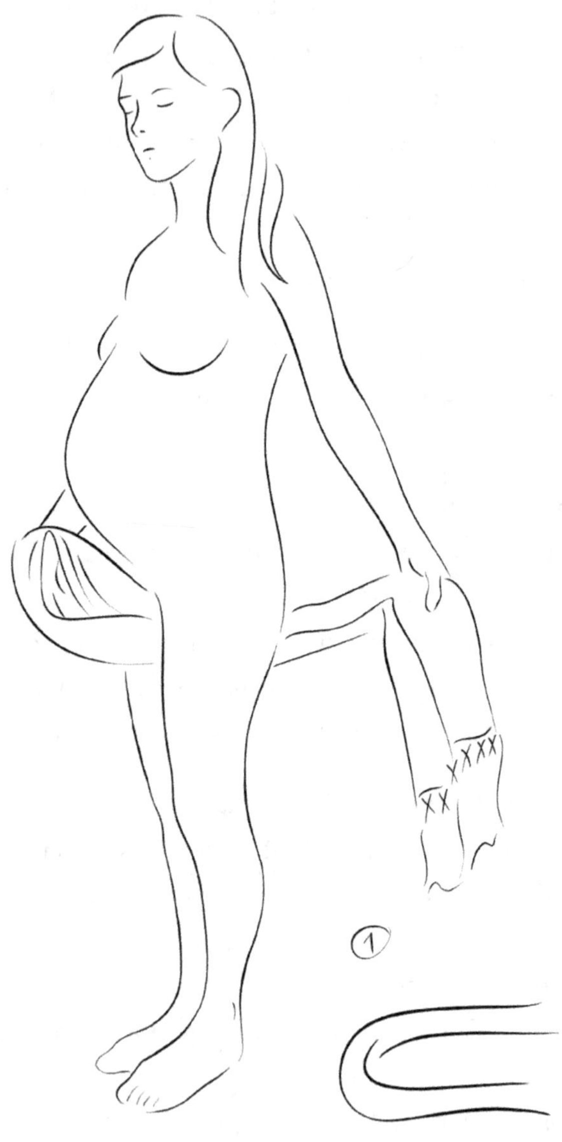

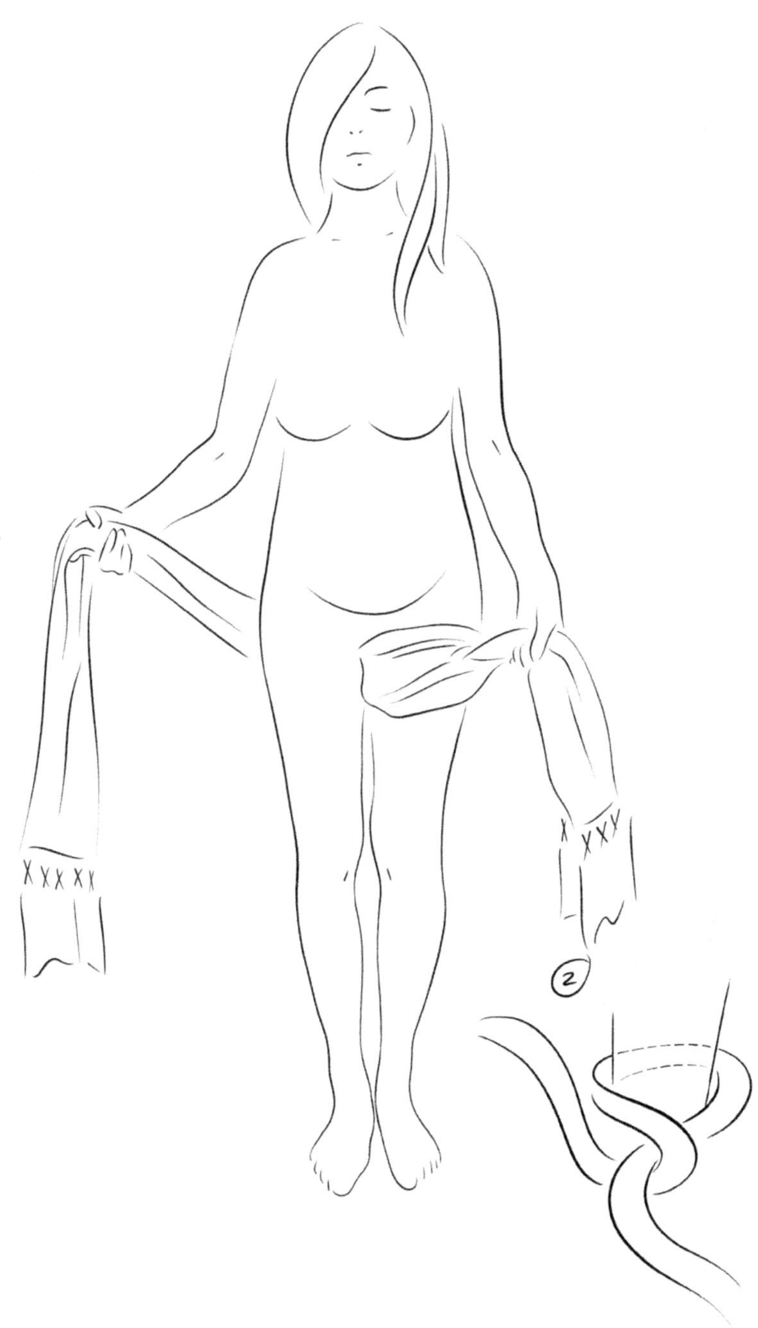

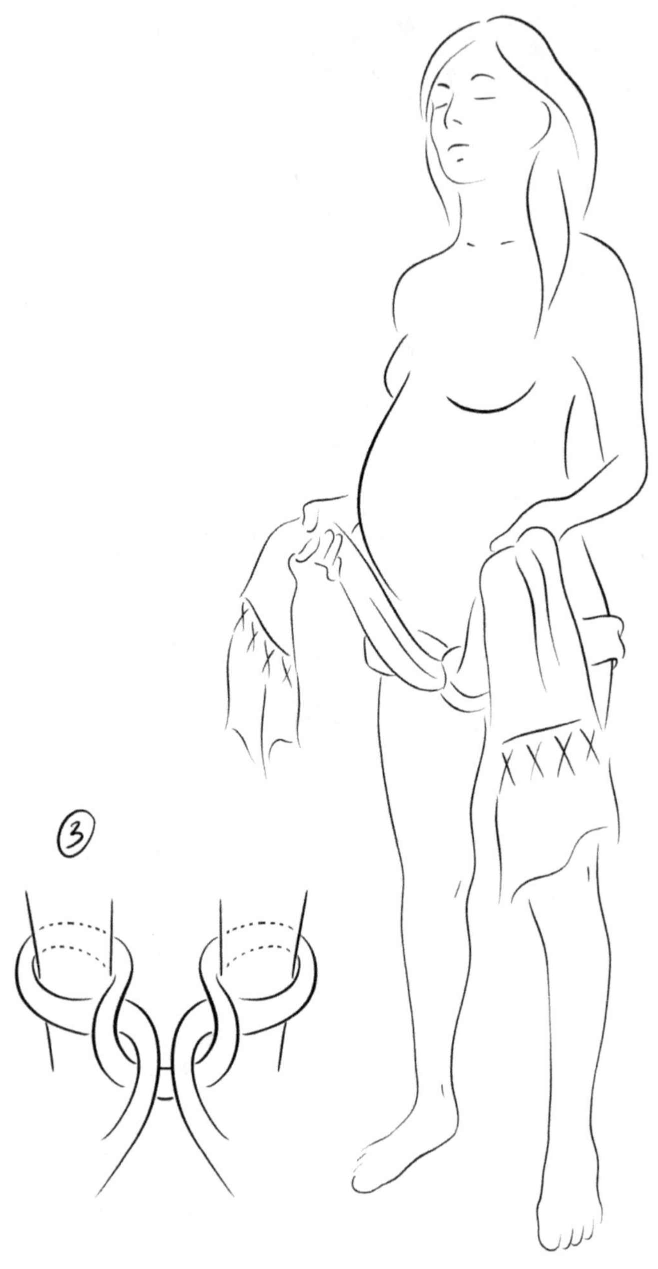

Ecaterina Mikitenko

In most cases, the aforementioned methods work, and if the mother and the baby feel well, it is possible to allow the body as much time as it needs for cervical dilation. **There is no need to rush if there are no risks to the mother or the baby.** Remember that childbirth is highly individual, and the range of normalcy is broader than we might think.

IF THINGS DON'T GO AS PLANNED DURING LABOR

My dear, I want to warn you that sometimes childbirth can deviate significantly from the planned course, even if you don't anticipate it. It happens!

There are situations where a mother strongly desires a natural birth and prepares for it, but interventions become necessary during labor. A mother might have believed that she could manage the pain on her own and give birth without epidural anesthesia, but then found it necessary for pain relief. Sometimes, a mother plans for a vaginal birth but ends up needing a cesarean section. Various circumstances can arise.

And I truly want you to know that if you prepare for childbirth during pregnancy, consciously choose your birth team and place, and act in alignment with yourself during labor, then **you have done everything within your**

control. The only thing you can do if labor doesn't go according to plan is to accept it and go with the flow. It's not your fault, because no matter how prepared you are for childbirth, it's a process where not everything depends on you.

There are forces that govern the order on our Earth, which control the processes of life and death on this planet. You can call them God, Creator, higher powers, nature, or destiny. It's not important. What matters is that you know there is something greater than you that guides your childbirth. Just agree with it and accept it. Trust in this 'greater' power and believe that what is happening is necessary, even if we don't immediately understand the purpose behind it.

There is also the concept of the soul's choice of the child. It is the choice of **how a person wants to come into this world**: the path, circumstances, conditions, and people they want to be surrounded by. How the birth process unfolds can significantly impact the baby's health, the formation of certain character traits, and the programming of behavior patterns in different life situations. This is studied in perinatal psychology, and if you're interested in it, I'm sure you'll find more information about it.

How a child is born largely shapes their life. Therefore, the soul's choice of the child carries more weight than your personal desire to have a particular birthing experience, and their choice may not align with your plan! You might be able to give birth as many times as you want, and have a chance to have a different experience, but your child can only be born once in their lifetime, and they have the right to choose their own script. You are merely their guide into this world.

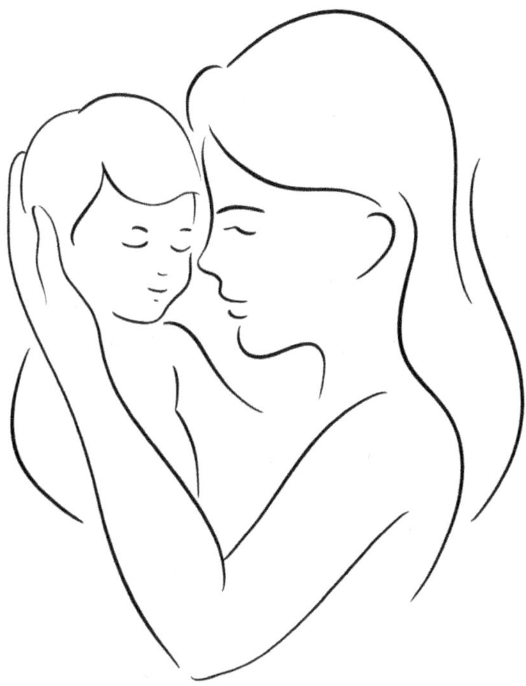

If something doesn't go as you want during your childbirth... just remember that **you are in labor for your child**. And if they have chosen you as their mother, it means that you are the one who can provide them with the experience their soul needs, including during birth.

FULL DILATION

When a woman reaches full or almost full dilation of the cervix (9-10 centimeters, also referred to as 'five fingers'), the transitional phase of labor begins. This is the time when the first stage of contractions ends and the second stage of pushing begins.

Contractions during this time are very frequent and intense, occurring every two minutes or even less. Sometimes they come one after another, with little to no breaks in between. Additionally, you may experience chills or hot flashes, nausea, and even vomiting, as well as trembling in your legs.

This is a challenging moment in childbirth, my dear. You may feel like you can't endure any longer. You might think you're dying. You may even beg for a cesarean section, even if it wasn't part of your plan, just to get it all over with. It's normal! Many women go through this. This 'weakness' doesn't mean that you are poorly prepared for childbirth or that you're not handling it well. It indicates that you are in the transition phase and are about to enter the pushing stage.

It would be wonderful if someone reminded you during these difficult moments that you are strong and that everything will soon pass. Once the pushing stage begins, all sensations will immediately change. The pain will diminish, and the desire to work hard to deliver your baby will emerge.

There's nothing special to do during the transitional phase (such as administering medications or intervening in any other way). It simply needs to be experienced. If you feel like roaring, roar. If you want to assume a strange position, do it. Forget about the fact that you were once a well-mannered, civilized woman! The transitional phase of labor is the time when all your **natural, animal power is unleashed**, when your brain shuts off, and wild instincts guide you. It's unlikely that you will ever experience anything like this outside of childbirth. It can be a very intriguing, even profound spiritual experience – if you are open to it.

The duration of the transition phase of labor can vary. Some women experience a transition period that lasts around 30 minutes, while for others it can extend to several hours. If the baby's condition is good, indicated by their heart rate, there is no need to rush the onset of pushing. The most ideal approach is to wait for the natural strong urge to push. Forcing pushing solely based on complete dilation is an aggressive and often traumatic tactic.

If the transitional period is significantly prolonged, and pushing does not begin, there may be reasons for this. One possible reason is a cervical lip, where a part of the cervix folds over the baby's head like a hood. The presence of a cervical lip is determined by the doctor or midwife during labor.

A cervical lip can be manually corrected by the midwife, or you can assist the cervix in correcting itself using certain positions:

1. Back-lying position with a roll under the sacrum: lie on your back and place a roll (such as a rolled-up towel) under your sacrum. Maintain this position for three contractions. It helps align the cervix properly, facilitating easier passage of the baby's head.

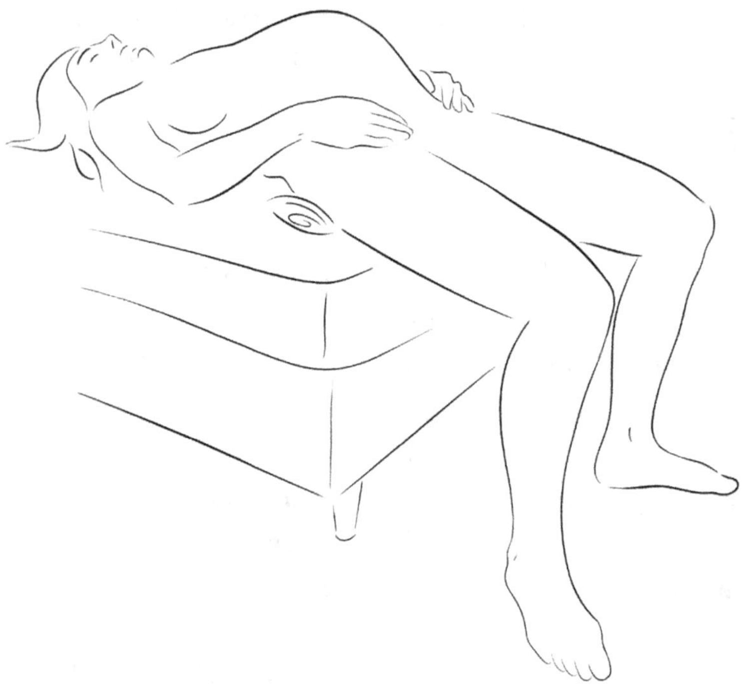

2. Hands-and-knees position, with the pelvis elevated above the head. It is effective to alternate between this position and lying on the roll.

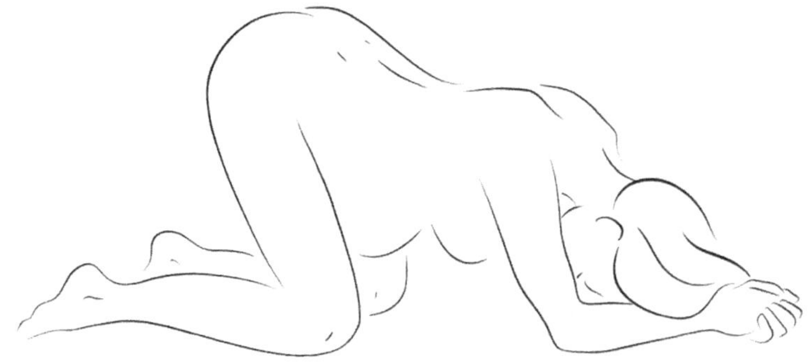

3. Rocking in a hands-and-knees position.

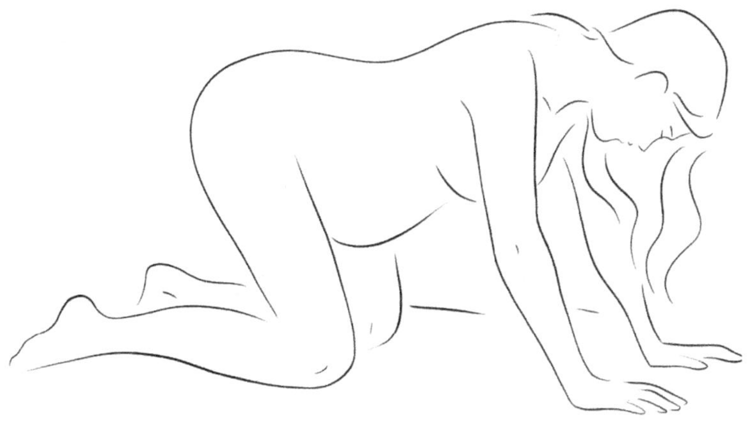

Another possible reason why pushing doesn't start despite complete dilation is that the baby's head hasn't descended. In such cases, shaking movements can be helpful.

1. Stand with your feet wide apart and try rocking back and forth, lifting your heels off the floor and tapping them on the ground. You can also make slow circular movements with your hips and torso.

2. Stand with your feet shoulder-width apart and gently shake your hips without lifting your feet off the floor (similar to a movement in Eastern dances). This movement, called *Come out, baby, come out*, is part of the Dancing For Birth™ childbirth preparation program.

3. Sit on a chair with your knees on either side of your partner, leaning your back against them. Ask your partner to hold you by the chest, while the midwife or doula rhythmically taps on your knees. This technique helps relax the pelvic floor muscles that may hinder the baby's descent. I learned about this method from midwife Anhelina Martinez, who uses it in her practice frequently.

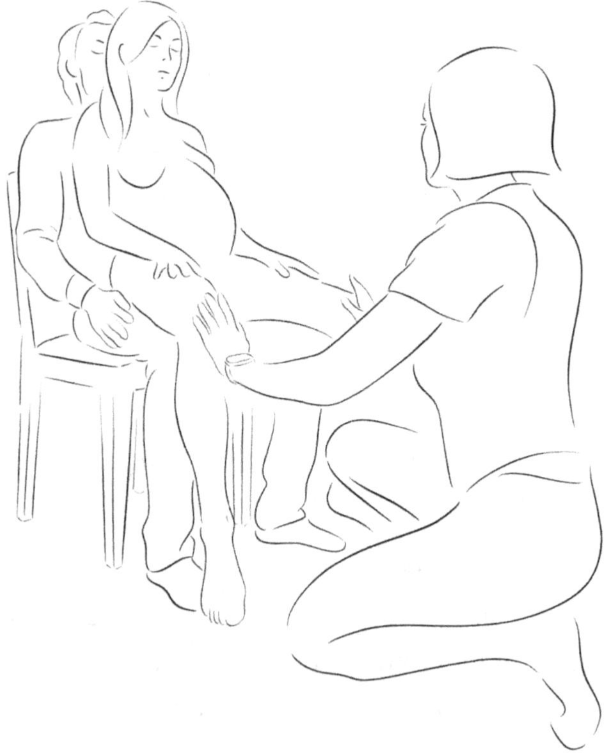

Ecaterina Mikitenko

PUSHING

Following the transitional period, the second stage of labor begins – pushing, or the passage of the baby through the birth canal. What do you need to know about this?

As I mentioned before, during the transitional period of labor, it is best to continue experiencing contractions until you feel the instinctive urge to push. It is similar to an overwhelming, intense desire to have a bowel movement. Once you feel this urge, you will have no doubts about what to do next, how to behave, or how to push correctly because your body will take over – it is a reflexive process known as the fetal ejection reflex. Trust your instincts and sensations in this moment!

There may be situations where you don't feel the urge to push, but are required to do so because your doctor or midwife instructs you to. If it is not possible to wait for natural urges to push, you will have to exert your own efforts to deliver the baby, as your body may not be fully prepared for it yet.

HOW TO PUSH

If you don't feel strong urges to push, it can be difficult to understand how to push correctly. One thing you should know is to engage your abdominal muscles and push 'down' rather than 'in your face'. A woman may exert a lot of effort during pushing, but if all the tension goes to her head, it is entirely ineffective. This can cause redness in the face and bursting of blood vessels in the eyes, but it won't help the baby move even a millimeter!

To understand what and how to tense during pushing, take a deep breath and hold it for a few seconds. While holding your breath, use your willpower to tense the lower abdomen, similar to how you might tense your abdomen to relieve constipation.

Remember this sensation: **how** you did it.

Here's the principle: when you have a contraction (because pushing involves the same uterine contractions but without pain), take a deep breath, tuck your chin to your chest, and begin a long, forceful exhale while strongly tensing your abdominal muscles and lower abdomen. Your exhale will be loud, with a sound resembling a growl or grunt. Please, don't be embarrassed by it.

> **During childbirth, you should never feel embarrassed about any natural expressions!**

This powerful pushing effort lasts for about 15-20 seconds, after which you quickly and deeply inhale air into your lungs and without pausing, start pushing again for about 20 seconds. Typically, a woman manages to do three pushes during one contraction. Once the contraction or push ends, relax and rest. You should only push during contractions.

POSITIONS FOR PUSHING

During pushing, your body will intuitively choose the most suitable position, just like during contractions. Therefore, stay mobile during the pushing phase.

Vertical positions are highly recommended for pushing:

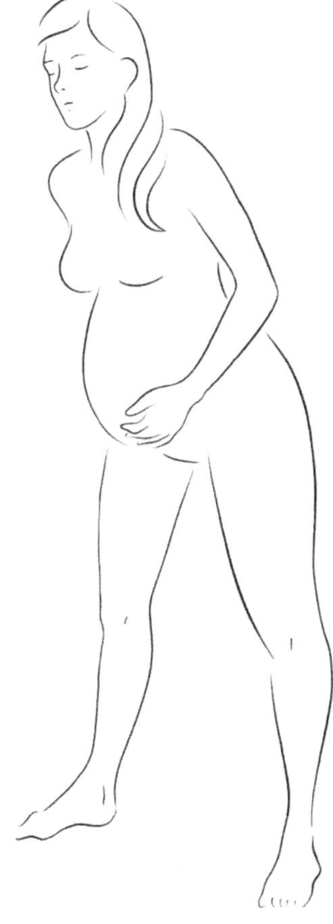

Standing

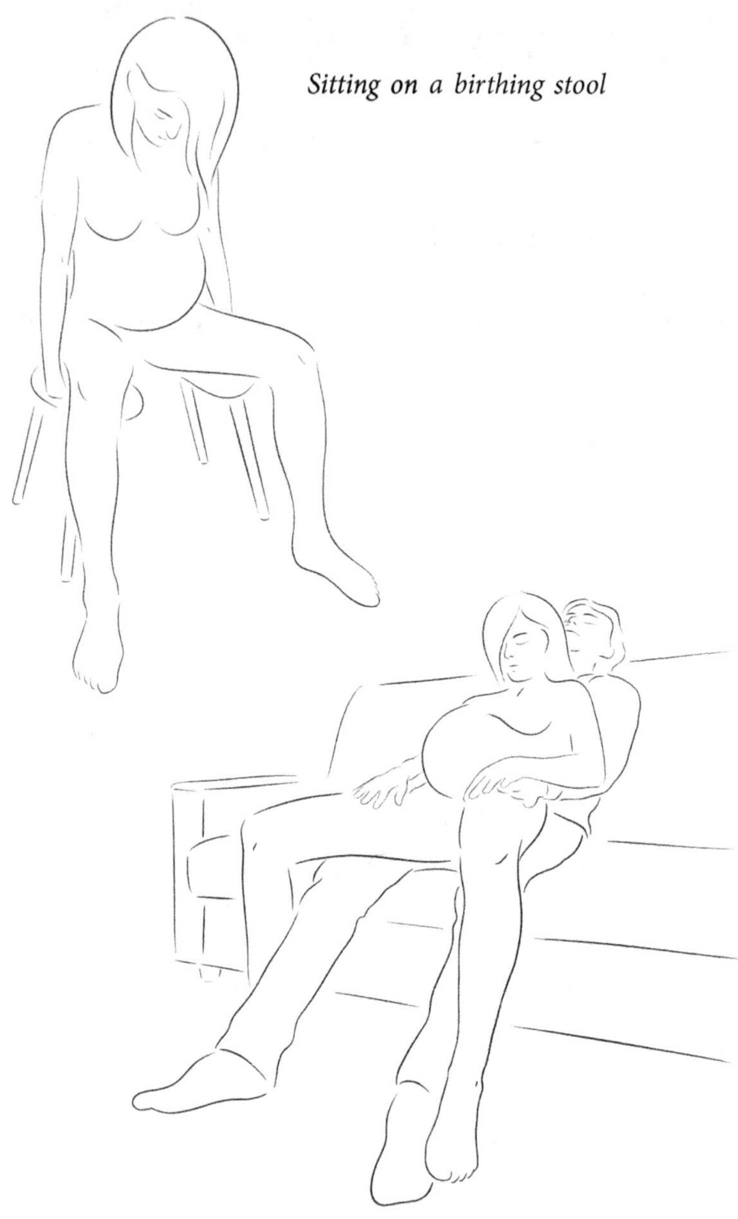

Sitting on a chair or seat on your partner's knees with your
legs wide apart and leaning your back against them

Ecaterina Mikitenko

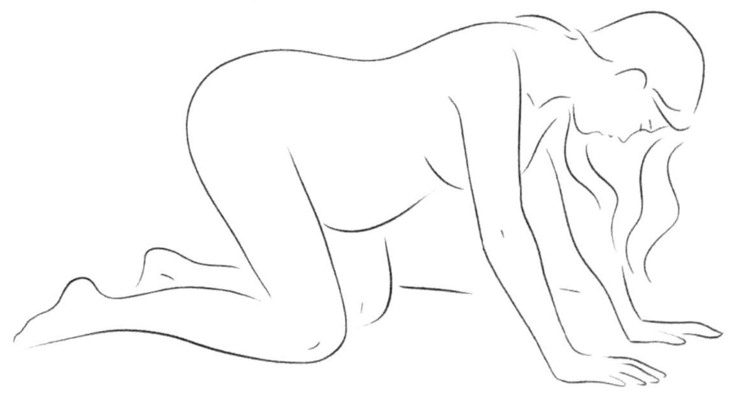

On all fours

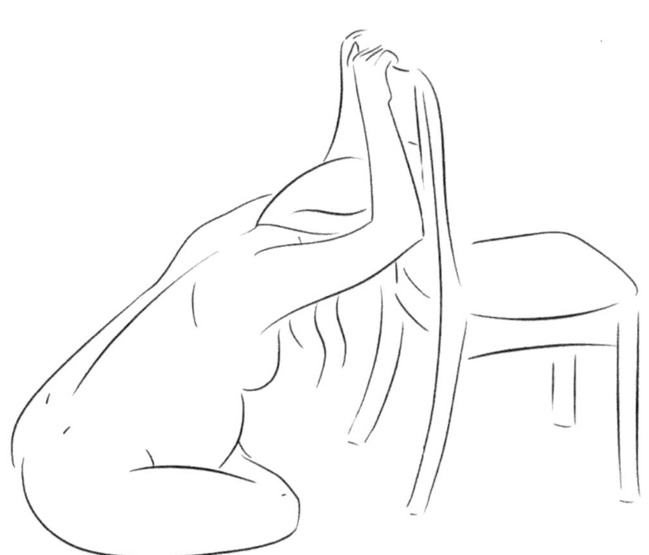

Kneeling on the floor, leaning your hands on the bed or chair

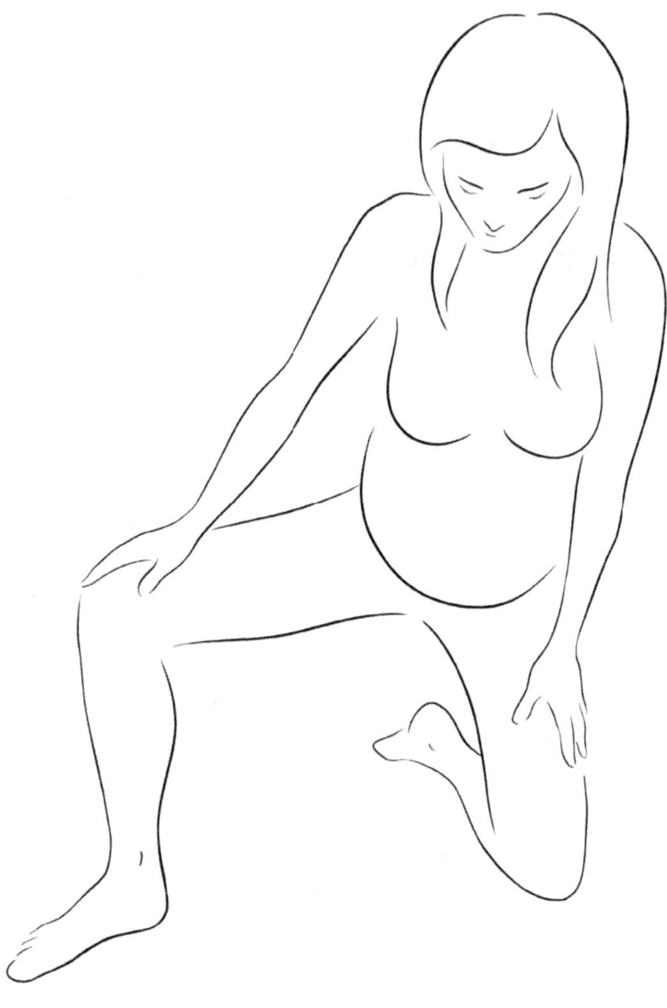

Asymmetric kneeling (one knee on the floor, the other foot planted on the floor and extended to the side)

Ecaterina Mikitenko

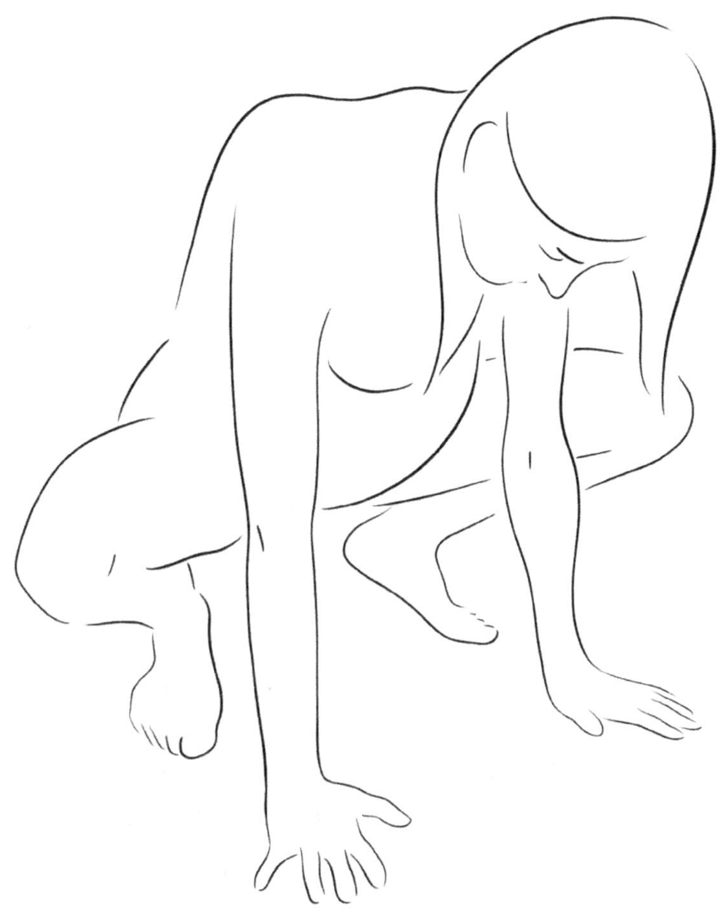

Squatting (best to practice these throughout pregnancy!).

Many studies indicate that vertical births help accelerate the pushing phase and facilitate easier delivery of the baby. And it's true because gravity plays a significant role. Remember, **gravity is your friend during childbirth**.

However, you may personally prefer a different position for pushing, such as lying on your side on the bed. Listen to your body! Do what feels right and **comfortable for you**.

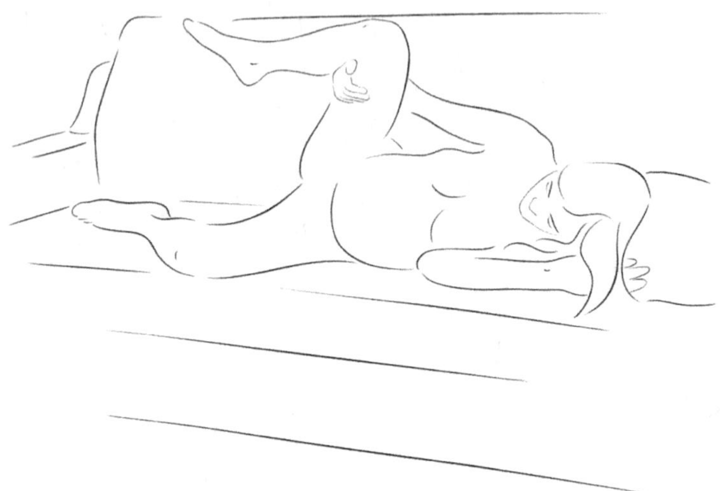

It's essential that the position you choose allows for movement of your pelvis. Why? Sometimes **a slight tilt of the pelvis forward or to the side can increase the internal space and release a few extra millimeters**, which can be critical for the baby's head to progress.

If the baby is moving slowly and having difficulty navigating through the birth canal, try creating asymmetry in your pelvis by gently rocking your hips from side to side. In the Dancing For Birth™ program, there is an exercise called *Mighty Mama* for this purpose. In a sumo wrestler-like position with a slightly forward-leaning torso, wide stance, and hands resting on the hips, we gracefully shift our weight from one leg to the other, swaying from side to side.

                                    Ecaterina Mikitenko

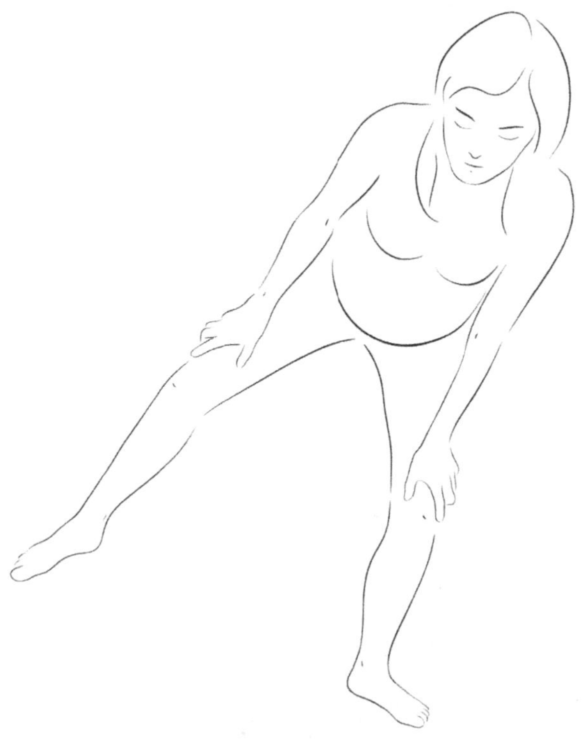

Unlike contractions, during pushing, **you should not be too active** or move around excessively. Furthermore, it is not recommended to walk during pushing, to avoid trapping the baby's head in the birth canal. If you need to move during the pushing phase, please do so with your legs wide apart to prevent any harm to the baby's head.

Also, remember that during pushing, **you should not sit on any surface** that creates pressure on the baby's head. You can only sit on a specialized birthing stool with a hole in the middle, where there is no pressure on the perineum.

THE RING OF FIRE

At some point, when the baby's head is close to emerging, it will start to appear through the vaginal opening. With each subsequent push, the baby's head will increasingly spread the labia and stretch the tissues of the perineum. This is normal.

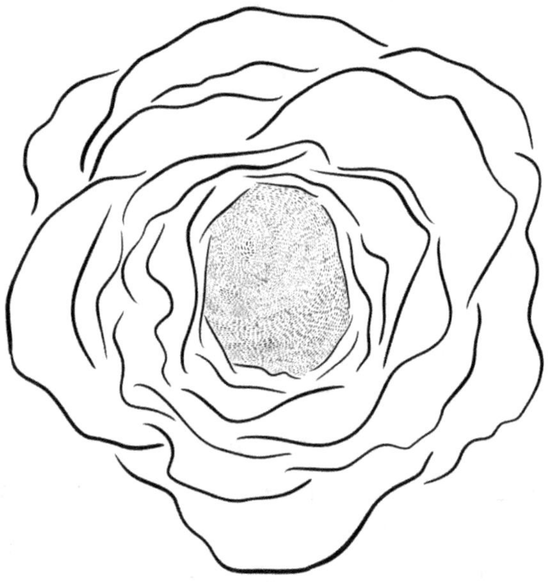

Pay close attention here. When the baby's head reaches its maximum diameter and spreads the labia wide apart, you will feel a strong burning sensation in the perineal area. It may feel like everything is about to tear and rupture. This is called the 'ring of fire', but don't be afraid. It will last for about a minute during a contraction. If you breathe correctly at this moment, you are likely to avoid tears.

    Ecaterina Mikitenko

What should you do if you feel the ring of fire? **Breathe like a dog** (panting) and don't push at all! Open your mouth, stick out your tongue, and breathe rapidly during the pushing phase without pushing at all. Try practicing this beforehand to understand how it feels.

The baby's head, aided by uterine contractions, will smoothly and gently slide through the perineum. Because the perineal tissues are stretched to their maximum, any additional effort on your part can lead to a complete tear. Unfortunately, during the ring of fire, you may have the strongest urge to push like never before. This desire can only be suppressed using the dog panting technique.

Once the baby's head is born, stop panting and return to your normal breathing. With one more push, you will see your baby.

BIRTH OF THE BABY

And here is your baby! He or she is born! Finally! What a joy! Whatever happened before this moment is now in the past. It's all over, and your long-awaited meeting has arrived!

Ask to have your little one placed on your chest right away, hold them close to you, and... **greet your baby!** Welcome them to the new world that they are seeing for the first time! Get to know your baby and say aloud how happy you are to meet them, as they have gone through a challenging journey, and it is essential for them to hear these words. He or she will remember them for a lifetime.

"Hello, baby! I'm your mom. How wonderful that you were born! How amazing that you exist and that you are who you are! I am so happy for you! I love you! I am here for you."

These few simple phrases are extremely important for **building trust in the world for the baby and creating a sense of security**. The feeling that *I am welcomed in this world* and that *I am good*.

Remember when I mentioned perinatal psychology? Well, the first 15 minutes after birth determine how a person will perceive this world and themselves in it in the future. It's **a subconscious program that is imprinted for a lifetime**. So, let it be a positive one for your baby!

Stay in skin-to-skin contact with your baby for as long as possible. The longer, the better. Ideally for two hours. If the baby is doing well and doesn't require any resuscitation measures, there's no rush. You both deserve rest. Weighing, dressing, and other procedures can wait.

Don't worry about the umbilical cord. After birth, it will continue to pulsate for some time (usually up to 20 minutes) because it allows the baby to receive necessary blood from the placenta. Ask for delayed cord clamping, preferably before the placenta is delivered. This way, the blood will not flow back from the baby to the placenta.

The baby won't experience pathological jaundice, and it won't provoke postpartum bleeding. It is safe!

BIRTH OF THE PLACENTA

The birth process is considered incomplete until the placenta is delivered. Unfortunately, according to the protocol for natural placental birth, only 30 minutes are allocated for this stage. For most women, the placenta detaches within 20-30 minutes after the baby's birth. However, for some women, it may take longer, and if there is no bleeding, it is possible to wait for the placenta to be delivered for a longer period.

If you encounter difficulties with the birth of the placenta, there can be two reasons:

1. The placenta has not fully or partially detached from the uterine wall.

2. The placenta has detached but cannot be delivered (it is stuck in the cervical canal or in the vagina).

HOW TO HELP THE PLACENTA TO BE DELIVERED

- **Create conditions necessary for birth (warmth, darkness, and quiet)**. For the placenta to be born, oxytocin is needed, and you already know what is needed for oxytocin. If you feel cold, ask for warm socks and covers. Drink a hot beverage (you can have hot water with honey and lemon). Relax. Admire your baby, enjoy bonding with them – during these processes, oxytocin is produced in large quantities.

- **Assume a vertical position** and stay in it for a while. Squatting is very convenient for delivering the placenta. Gravity in this case helps, just like during the baby's birth.

- **Attach the baby to the breast**. Nipple stimulation is a highly effective way to stimulate uterine contractions. If the baby is tired after birth and doesn't want to suckle, try gently stimulating the nipples with your fingers.

- **Cough**. Coughing greatly increases intra-abdominal pressure, which can help expel the placenta. You can also try blowing into an empty bottle. Ideally, be in a squatting position or sit on a birthing stool.

- **Try to induce a gag reflex**. Surprisingly, it works! This may be due to the hormone acetylcholine, which is produced during vomiting and during contractions.

What should you not do? Do not pull on the umbilical cord. If the placenta has not fully detached, pulling on it will detach a piece of the placenta from the uterine wall, which can lead to severe postpartum bleeding!

May everything go well in your birth, my dear! I wish it with every fiber of my being!

PART TWO

AFTER CHILDBIRTH

And you also deserve rest, care, and support to recover your body, which has done significant work in carrying and giving birth to your baby. Please know that you need to recover after childbirth. Please understand that you have the right to do so. Please believe that you are worthy of it. For your physical health. For your psychological well-being. For your self-esteem. Believe it and try to organize a well-planned postpartum period for yourself. I will be your guide in this, my dear.

YOUR RECOVERY

Can you imagine the amount of work your body has gone through during childbirth? How many of its resources it has expended? And before that, how many resources were dedicated to building your baby's body, brick by brick, during pregnancy!

Over the course of nine months, changes in your body occurred gradually. Your uterus grew, internal organs shifted. Your posture changed to create balance for your growing belly, your center of gravity shifted, and dynamic patterns in your brain (habits of performing certain actions without thinking) were altered. Your body gave its best to support the growth and development of your baby.

And now that baby is born. Everything in your body has changed, in an instant:

- Intra-abdominal pressure dropped sharply.

- The abdominal cavity suddenly had a lot of space.

- All internal organs remained shifted.

- Due to the hormone relaxin (which was necessary during pregnancy and childbirth), all ligaments and joints became very weak.

- An open wound formed inside the uterus after the placenta detached.

- Soft tissues were traumatized after the passage of the baby through them.

- The uterus was greatly stretched.

- The body lost about half a liter of blood during childbirth and will lose the same amount in the next forty days as the uterus contracts and cleanses itself...

Your body is weakened and injured, quite literally. It needs to heal and regain strength. This requires time (typically around forty days), energy and resources, as well as knowledge of how to support your body.

Recovery guidelines after vaginal and cesarean births differ slightly, so as I describe each principle, I will make a note of these differences where applicable.

The first and simplest thing you can give your body is **bed rest**. Do you know what the midwife and postpartum recovery specialist Alena Lebedeva says? The number of days you need to observe bed rest after childbirth is equal to the number of births you have had. If it's your first birth, you should lie in bed without getting up for one day. For the second birth, lie in bed for two days. For the third birth, three days, and so on. This is the minimum, but you can do it for longer if you feel the need.

There is also a wise saying about the first forty days after childbirth, or rather how you should spend that time. The first week, stay in bed; the second week, stay on the bed; the third week, stay near the bed; and the fourth week, stay close to the bed.

Jokes aside, that's how it is: for the first four to six weeks (!) after vaginal birth and the first two weeks after a cesarean section, you should lie down, rest, and recover as much as possible. Don't stand at the stove, don't clean the floors, don't prepare for hosting guests on the third day after birth, don't walk around the neighborhood or park pushing a stroller. You need to lie down. Take care of yourself.

You know why? Because the potential consequences of early verticalization after childbirth (when a woman starts spending too much time in an upright position too soon) can be quite unpleasant. These consequences include organ prolapse and descent (bladder, uterus, vaginal walls), hemorrhoids, urinary incontinence, digestive system disorders, urinary and reproductive system issues, back pain, spinal misalignment in the thoracic and lumbar regions (sunken chest and protruding abdomen, also known as 'pregnancy sail'), and spinal disc protrusions.

During the time you will be lying down (at least for the first week or the first few days), the hormone relaxin (which weakened your muscles and ligaments) will be eliminated from your body. The ligaments and joints will strengthen, the pelvic floor muscles will strengthen, and there will be a realignment of the internal organs, as well as a change in the dynamic stereotype.

Please, spend several days resting in bed, even if you feel energetic and full of strength (which often happens after easy deliveries). Ask your loved ones to take care of you, at least for the first few days after the baby's birth. Or better yet, provide you with assistance and support throughout the first month after childbirth.

If you had a cesarean section, it is also important for you to lie down for the first two or three days after the surgery and spend a significant amount of time in bed during the first two weeks. To prevent adhesion formation and thrombus

*formation, it is beneficial to engage in gentle
stretching and breathing exercises while lying in
bed. I will tell you more about this later.*

*After two weeks following a cesarean birth, you
can and should gradually incorporate more
activity into your life, including light walks for
short distances. Wearing an abdominal belt,
a specialized postoperative (not postpartum!)
bandage, or using fabric to support your
abdomen, will be helpful for supporting the
internal organs. I will provide more information
on this as well.*

WHAT TO DO WHILE YOU SPEND A LOT OF TIME IN BED AFTER CHILDBIRTH

While you'll be spending a lot of time in bed during the first weeks after childbirth, you can find plenty of engaging activities to keep yourself entertained and make your postpartum recovery more interesting. Otherwise, you may feel tempted to get up and find something to do!

During the first month after childbirth, a newborn sleeps for 18-20 hours a day, so you'll have plenty of time for yourself! Consider what you'd like to do during the postpartum period. Here are a few ideas:

Reading books

There are so many useful and worthwhile books for parents available now! I'll share with you a short list of books on children's health, parenting, and motherhood. Hopefully, you'll find something useful from this list:

- Galina Filippova, *Psychology of Motherhood*

- Donald Winnicott, *The Child and the Family*

- Yulia Gippenreiter, *Communicating with Children. How?*

- Ludmila Petranovskaya, *Secret Support: Attachment in a Child's Life*

- Janusz Korczak, *Loving a Child*

- Masaru Ibuka, *After Three, It's Too Late*

- Gordon Neufeld, *Hold On to Your Kids*

- Lena Danilova, *Encyclopedia of Developmental Games*

- Ilya Arshavsky, *Your Child. At the Origins of Health*

- Evgeny Komarovsky, *The Beginning of Your Child's Life*

- William, Martha, Robert and James Sears, *The Baby Book: Everything You Need to Know About Your Baby from Birth to Age Two*

- Olga Gofman, *Mom-Doctor. Why Do Our Children Get Sick?*

- Robert Mendelsohn, *How to Raise a Healthy Child in Spite of Your Doctor*

- Ingrid Bauer, *Diaper-Free: The Gentle Wisdom of Natural Infant Hygiene*

- Diane Wiessinger, Diana West, and Teresa Pitman, *The Womanly Art of Breastfeeding*

Online learning

In addition to books, the modern market offers a multitude of educational courses, seminars, and programs. The online format is very convenient – you can learn about what interests you from experts all over the world, all while lying in your own bed: nutrition, art therapy, photography, editing, foreign languages, psychosomatics, psychology, painting, singing, and much more. Choose what you specifically enjoy.

Movie watching

If you love movies, now is the perfect time to indulge in them because the next opportunity to watch a movie may not come soon!

Crafts and creativity

Engaging in creative activities helps prevent postpartum depression, so it's a good idea to include it in your list of hobbies. You can conveniently use ready-made craft kits (such as stress-relief coloring books, sequin mosaics, embroidery, and more), or you can simply draw or create with any artistic materials that inspire you.

Acquiring a new profession

Perhaps after giving birth, you might want to learn a new profession. It's entirely possible! There are professions that can be learned online in just two or three months. In the realm of parenthood, these could include becoming a professional doula, postpartum doula, breastfeeding consultant, or sleep consultant. Your experience with childbirth and motherhood might inspire you to help other women.

BELLY BINDING

When you start getting out of bed more often than just for bathroom or shower purposes, to avoid the unpleasant consequences of early verticalization, it's important for you to learn how to bind your belly with fabric to provide support to your internal organs and muscles. This is the second important principle of postpartum recovery. There are different methods of belly binding, and one of them will surely suit you.

> *If you had a cesarean section, it is also necessary for you to bind your belly. An alternative is to use a special postoperative (not postpartum) abdominal binder. Why should you bind your belly? While your pelvic floor muscles have suffered less compared to vaginal childbirth,*

everything else regarding changes in your body and the consequences of verticalization are just as relevant to you as they are to a woman who gave birth vaginally. When binding your belly, make sure that no knots from the fabric come into contact with the incision area. And always place a soft, breathable lining between the incision and the fabric used for binding.

It is very convenient to use special tools for belly binding after childbirth, such as a bengkung, binder, or faja. Describing these methods in a book is quite challenging, so I suggest you watch instructional videos on YouTube while you observe bed rest and have plenty of free time!

If you find it difficult to purchase or rent belly binding tools, I propose a simpler solution using materials that you most likely have at home:

Belly binding with a shawl

Take the longest shawl you have. Fold it lengthwise so that the width is about 25-30cm. Lie on your back and bend your legs at the knees. If you gave birth vaginally, prepare your belly for binding (lightly stroke your belly several times from the pubic bone to the navel, and then make a few circular massage motions clockwise).

Take the fabric, find the center, and place it at the bottom of your belly, covering the pubic area and hip bones. Lift your pelvis, bring the ends of the fabric to the back and tie a knot behind your back – try to tighten it around your thighs. Then bring the remaining ends forward and secure them by tucking them under the fabric snugly against your belly. You now have a supportive pocket for your belly.

To stand up, roll onto your side, push off with your elbow from the bed, and gently rise. This method of getting up will allow you to avoid straining your weak abdominal and pelvic floor muscles.

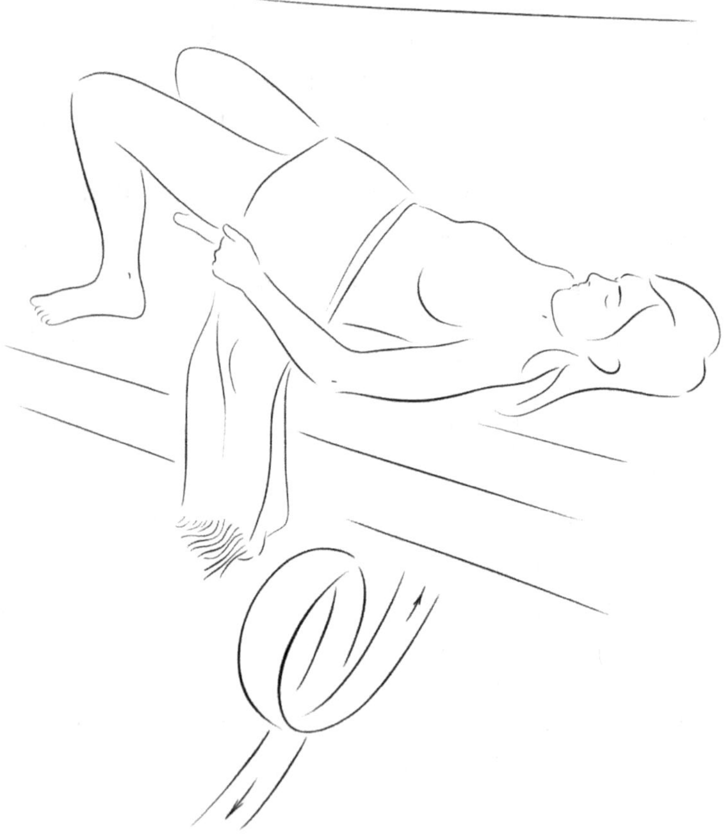

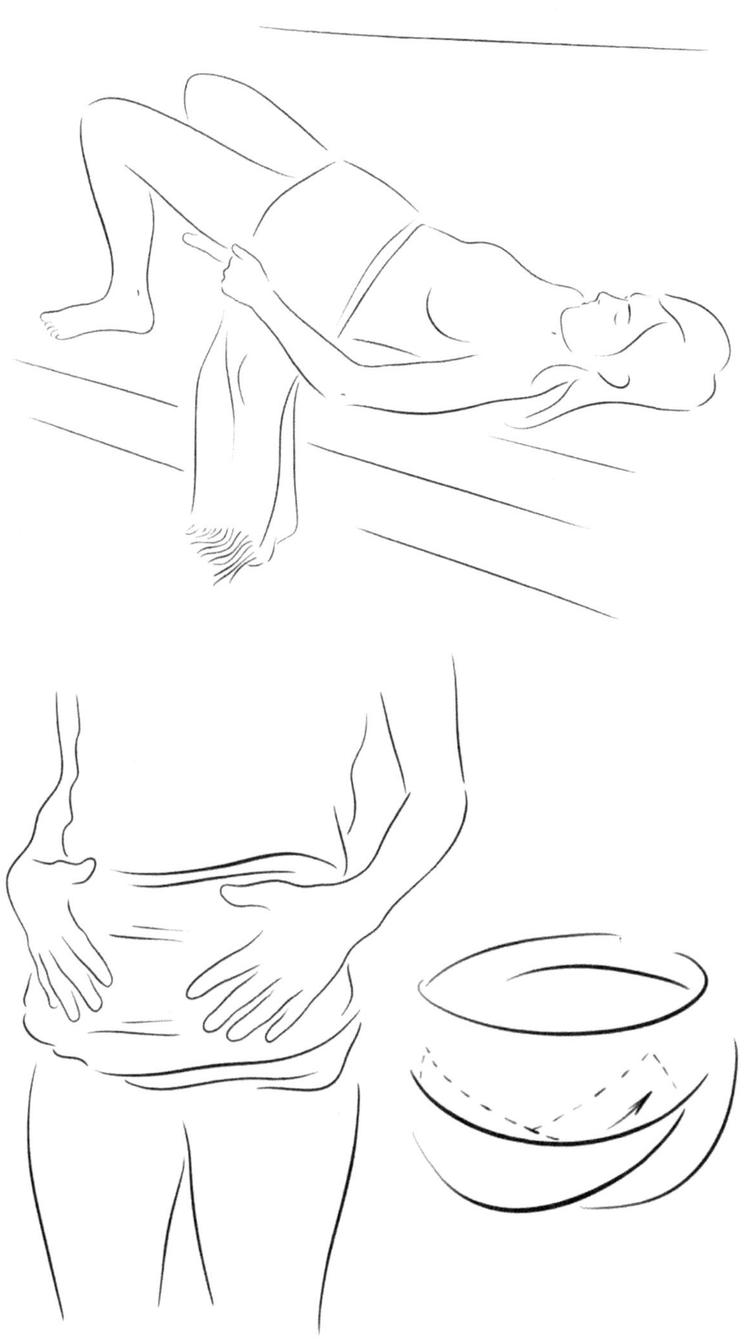

Belly binding with an old sheet, sling scarf, or 2-3 meter fabric strip

Fold the fabric lengthwise so that its width covers the distance from the middle of your ribs (under the bust line) to the upper third of your thigh. Find the center of the fabric, place it against your body at the front, and lie on your back with your knees bent and your hips raised. Bring the ends of the fabric behind your back.

Cross the fabric behind your back at the level of your hips and pull on the ends to tighten it around your thighs. Then bring the ends forward and tie them in a knot at the bottom of your belly, to the side of your pubic bone.

> *If you had a cesarean section, tie the knot on your thigh instead of near the pubic area.*

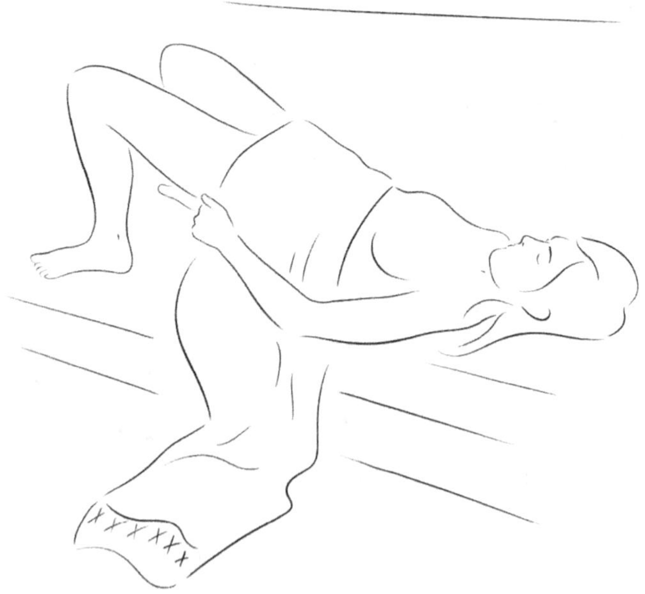

Ecaterina Mikitenko

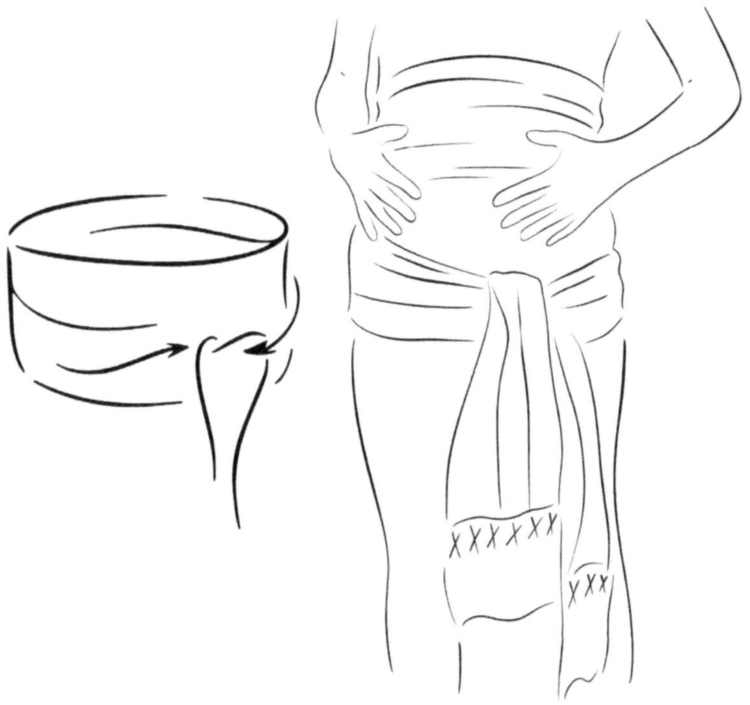

If you gave birth vaginally, it's helpful to prepare your belly with a gentle self-massage before binding. When getting up from the bed after binding, it's recommended to do so through your side. Once you're standing, check how snugly the fabric fits around your hips. If it's not tight enough, tighten it further.

Important: bind your belly only when you need to get up. Remove the binding fabric when you return to bed.

The methods I described using a shawl or a long fabric strip are suitable for the early days after childbirth when you get up infrequently and briefly. However, when you spend most of your time in an upright position, a bengkung, faja, or postpartum belly wrap will provide better support to your internal organs. If you don't have those, continue to bind with the available means. Ideally, you should do this for the first forty days after giving birth. Your body will thank you for it and repay you with improved health and well-being.

THE FIRST HOURS AFTER CHILDBIRTH

Now that you know the two main principles of postpartum recovery, let's return to where we left off in the first part of the book: your baby is born, the placenta is delivered, and your labor is over. The early postpartum period has begun.

The biggest danger during this period is the risk of postpartum hemorrhage. That's why the doctor or midwife will closely monitor you during this time. I'll share with you two recipes from experienced midwives that help the uterus contract better and **prevent excessive bleeding in the early postpartum period.**

Recipe for fenugreek drink

Ingredients

- Water – 1 cup
- Fenugreek – 1 tsp
- Ginger – to taste
- Lemon
- Honey
- Raspberry leaves (optional) – 1 tsp
- Orange (for flavor, optional) – 1 slice

Pour boiling water over all the ingredients except honey and let it steep for 10-20 minutes. Add honey to the drink when the water cools slightly.

Recipe for herbal tea

Ingredients

- Water – 1 cup
- Mixed herbs (nettle, yarrow, shepherd's purse) – 1 tbsp each
- Dried ginger – a pinch
- Honey
- Lemon

Pour boiling water over the herbs and ginger and let it steep for 10-20 minutes. When the tea cools slightly, add honey and lemon.

In the first hours after childbirth, you may experience various unusual sensations. This is normal! Stay calm and don't worry if you suddenly feel:

- **Tremors.** You may feel shaky or cold. This is due to a drop in arterial and intra-abdominal pressure. To help yourself, try to warm up. Put on warm socks, bundle up, and **drink something hot** or warm.

- **Painful uterine contractions.** If this is your first childbirth, you may not even feel the postpartum contractions. However, during second or subsequent births, the pain from these contractions can be very intense, similar to labor contractions. You can alleviate the pain in several ways:

  1. Self-massage of the abdomen with essential oils such as lavender, frankincense, or Roman chamomile. Mix one drop of essential oil with one teaspoon of a carrier oil (preferably warmed in a water bath) and gently massage your abdomen. You should experience relief relatively quickly.

  2. Apply warmth to your abdomen. This can be a warm cloth, a heating pad, or simply placing your hands on your abdomen and holding them there for a few minutes.

  3. Drink herbal tea made from hawthorn, motherwort, or fenugreek.

- **Unable to urinate.** In the first hours after childbirth, you may experience difficulties with urination. This is because the bladder can be swollen, and for the first 12-18 hours, you may find it challenging to empty your bladder. However, it is essential to urinate regularly because a full bladder hinders the uterus from contracting effectively. To help with urination, sit comfortably on the toilet and try to relax. If that doesn't work, you can try pouring warm water over your perineum using a plastic bottle. This can be helpful. Alternatively, you can turn on the tap to stimulate the urge to urinate. If you're unable to empty your bladder, please discuss the possibility of having a catheter inserted with your healthcare provider. Sometimes, it's the only way to relieve the accumulated urine.

- **Burning and pain in the perineum.** Even if you didn't tear during childbirth, there may be microcracks and tissue swelling that can cause discomfort and burning sensations. If you did tear, the pain from the tears adds to the discomfort. This is normal, and over time, the swelling and pain will decrease. To help yourself, make sure to thoroughly cleanse the area with warm water after each trip to the toilet. It's even better if you can use soothing herbal infusions such as chamomile, calendula, or oak bark. I will provide more details on how to care for the perineum after childbirth in the next section: *How to help your body heal.*

- **Severe weakness, dizziness.** Feeling weak and dizzy is common due to blood loss and decreased blood pressure. Drinking sweet, hot beverages with honey and lemon (water, tea, dried fruit compote, berry infusions) and consuming hot liquid food (a cup of bone broth or a small bowl of chicken soup) can help restore your strength and make you feel better.

Remember, my dear, that the first hours after childbirth lay the foundation for your proper postpartum recovery. Here's what you need to do during this time and the following forty days:

1. Help the uterus contract effectively.

2. Aid the body in healing.

3. Begin to restore blood.

HOW TO HELP THE UTERUS CONTRACT

Your uterus weighed about 60 grams before pregnancy. After childbirth, it weighs one kilogram! Can you imagine how much this muscular organ needs to contract in order to recover? And most of the work is done by the uterus in the first nine days. It starts immediately after childbirth. Let's create the best conditions for your uterus to contract:

Warmth

And I'll start talking to you about oxytocin again. What can we do, it's very important for us even after childbirth, especially for recovery! Of course, silence and darkness are also valuable after childbirth, but warmth is particularly important. So please, warm yourself up right after childbirth and continue to keep warm for all forty days.

- Warm your feet with woolen socks.

- Wrap yourself in a blanket or quilt.

- Drink a warm or slightly hot beverage (remember, I asked you to prepare it at the beginning of childbirth? The recipes for herbal tea, postpartum infusions, broth, and other drinks will be detailed below).

- Add one of the warming spices to your postpartum drink: dried ginger, rosemary, red pepper, or turmeric.

- Eat something warm, such as a restorative postpartum soup (recipe below).

In the past, after childbirth, women were always given an ice pack... on their stomachs. It was believed that this constricted blood vessels and reduced postpartum bleeding. But in reality, such a 'compress' only harms women and can have a negative impact on their reproductive health in the long run. There are other mechanisms at work during childbirth. So, if you need to put something on your stomach after childbirth, it should only be warmth.

Emptying the bladder

Our uterus is located between the bladder and the intestines. It lies behind the bladder, and if the bladder is full, it presses against the uterus and hinders its contractions. Therefore, it's important to regularly urinate after childbirth. Remember that due to the swelling of the bladder, you may experience difficulties with urination. Moreover, you may not feel the urge to urinate, even when the bladder is full. Simply go to the bathroom on a schedule (every two to three hours) and try to urinate. I have mentioned how to help yourself with this, but I'll repeat it here: sit comfortably on the toilet and try to relax. If it's difficult, you can try pouring warm water on your perineum from a plastic bottle. This can help. Alternatively, you can simply turn on the tap to stimulate the urge to urinate.

Lying on your back

You already know that after childbirth you need to lie down. But how should you lie down? It matters. In order for the uterus to contract better in the first few hours after childbirth, it's best to lie on your back. When a woman lies on her stomach after childbirth, the uterus 'sags' forward, in front of the bladder, and because of this 'bending', it contracts less effectively. The same thing happens when lying on your side: the uterus leans to one side. Try to lie on your back on the first day after childbirth. Later on, you can choose other positions.

Breastfeeding

When you breastfeed your baby, the hormone oxytocin is released, which helps the uterus contract. Breastfeed your baby as often as possible after childbirth. This will not only help the uterus but also facilitate the timely arrival of milk.

Black seed oil

This is a very beneficial product for postpartum recovery as it helps the uterus contract better and enhances lactation. However, it should be consumed in small doses. Mix one teaspoon of black seed oil with one teaspoon of honey and consume it after a meal. **Please do not exceed this dosage.**

Cinnamon

This spice, like black seed oil, strengthens uterine contractions. You can add a small pinch of cinnamon to tea, compote, and even food (cinnamon porridge is very delicious).

Uterine point

There are situations where a few days after childbirth, a woman's discharge becomes very scanty or stops altogether. This is not normal! One possible reason for this is a retroverted uterus, which causes the discharge to stagnate inside. In this case, a method that I learned from midwife Alyona Lebedeva may help you. Locate the uterine point at the bottom of your abdomen. It is one-third of the distance from the pubic bone to the navel (closer to the pubic bone). Join your index and middle fingers and place them vertically on this point. Do not press! Just hold your fingers there until they naturally 'sink' inside. If this happens, it means your finger has entered the space between the uterus and the bladder. Thanks to this 'adjustment', the uterus will straighten, and the discharge will resume.

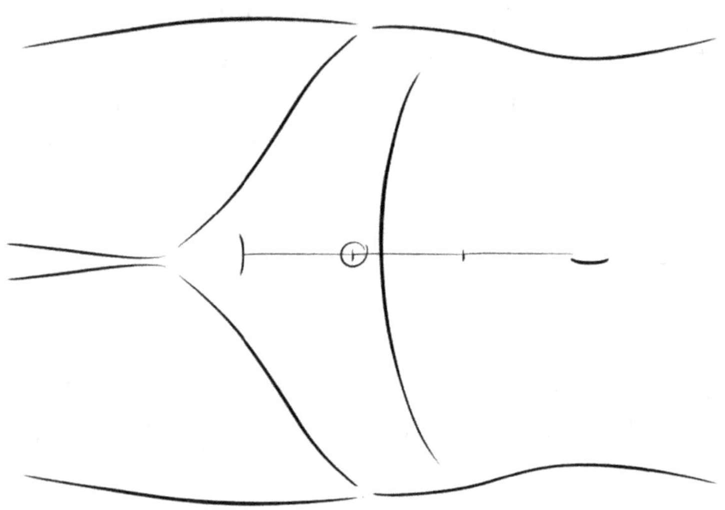

HOW TO HELP YOUR BODY HEAL

By resting, lying down, and getting adequate sleep after childbirth, you are already assisting your body in its recovery and healing process. Now let's talk about what else you can do.

Appreciate your body

Your body has done tremendous work! It carried and delivered your baby! Even if you had a cesarean section,

Ecaterina Mikitenko

your body still brought your little one into this world. Say *"thank you"* to your body. Speak these words every day, feeling the love and gratitude in every fiber of your being for your beautiful, magical organism.

You can place your hands on your uterus, feel the warmth of your hands spreading throughout your body, and gently caress your belly. Give your body a little bit of your attention. It will respond beautifully to such care and love. And truly, it will make your postpartum recovery much more effective and easier.

Even if, initially, for some reason, you don't feel grateful towards your body, simply say *"thank you"*. One day, your feelings will change, and your words will become sincere.

Nourish your body

Your body needs high-quality restorative nutrition after childbirth because it lost many micronutrients during pregnancy and a significant amount of blood during delivery. Furthermore, after giving birth, it continues to provide the best for your baby through breastfeeding. If you don't eat with consideration for replenishing all the deficits, you can easily develop chronic anemia, and other health problems.

In the next section, where I discuss how to restore blood after childbirth, I will provide you with detailed information on restorative nutrition and will share several useful recipes for nourishing food. Read *Restorative beverage recipes* for even more.

Care for the perineum

The perineum always experiences trauma during vaginal childbirth. After all, it's no joke to pass a baby weighing 2-4kg through it! Even if there are no obvious tears or episiotomies, there are bound to be microcracks, abrasions and swelling.

How to care for the perineum

- After every visit to the toilet, cleanse with warm water or an infusion of antiseptic herbs. Chamomile and calendula reduce inflammation, St. John's wort and oak bark promote healing, and calendula also reduces swelling.

- If possible, avoid using postpartum pads or diapers. Lie on a disposable sheet and allow your perineum to be exposed to air.

- Apply warm compresses of cotton fabric soaked in a decoction of wound-healing herbs (calendula, St. John's wort, oak bark, chamomile) to the affected tissues every day.

- If you have tears or an episiotomy, avoid spreading your legs wide during the first few days. When you go to the toilet, take small, gentle steps. It's advisable to wrap a rebozo, scarf, or piece of fabric around your thighs to support your steps.

- If you have tears or an episiotomy, you can use special ointments and gels such as Solcoseryl (promotes rapid and effective wound healing), Traumeel, and Rescue.

Consult with your doctor or midwife before using them. Also, avoid sitting or standing for long periods until the stitches have healed. These positions exert pressure on the pelvic floor muscles and your injured perineum due to the force of gravity.

Remember to consult with your healthcare provider for personalized advice and guidance regarding your specific situation.

Help improve digestion

After childbirth, many women experience difficulties with bowel movements. This can be due to the displacement of the intestines and hormonal changes during pregnancy, weak peristalsis, or even psychological factors.

The first time you feel the need to have a bowel movement is usually around the third day after childbirth. This is normal. However, after that, make sure to maintain regular and soft bowel movements. Avoid constipation at all costs!

If you're experiencing difficulties with bowel movements, the following tips can help improve digestion:

- Drink an adequate amount of water (the recommended amount while breastfeeding is two and a half liters per day).

- Avoid consuming raw vegetables, fruits, and kefir (these foods may not help alleviate constipation after childbirth and can even worsen it).

- Include liquid and semi-liquid foods in your diet (soups and pureed porridges).

- Incorporate spices such as turmeric, cumin, and ginger into your meals and postpartum drinks.

- Consume bone broths (they help restore intestinal microflora).

- Eat baked apples.

- Include boiled beets in your diet.

- Consume prunes and raisins, and compote made from them.

- Perform circular clockwise strokes on your abdomen to promote digestion.

If you had a cesarean section, improving digestion is also important for you. You can follow all the recommendations mentioned above. Just remember that the massaging strokes should only be applied to the upper area from the ribs to the navel. You can start practicing them from the second day after the operation.

Self-massage

While you will be lying down during the first few days after giving birth, try to perform self-massage on your hands, thighs, and head. Massage your body to improve blood circulation.

- Several times a day, engage in gentle exercises: clench and unclench your fist, make circular motions with your hands, move your feet in different directions, stretch your shoulder joints, and massage your chest and collarbone area.

> *In the case of a cesarean section, this is even more important. To prevent the formation of blood clots and adhesions, start doing light exercises while lying in bed as early as four to six hours after the surgery, repeating them several times a day. Make sure not to get dizzy during the exercises. If that happens, stop immediately.*

- Smooth out your sides. I borrowed this exercise (along with the next one) from Alona Lebedeva. It will help

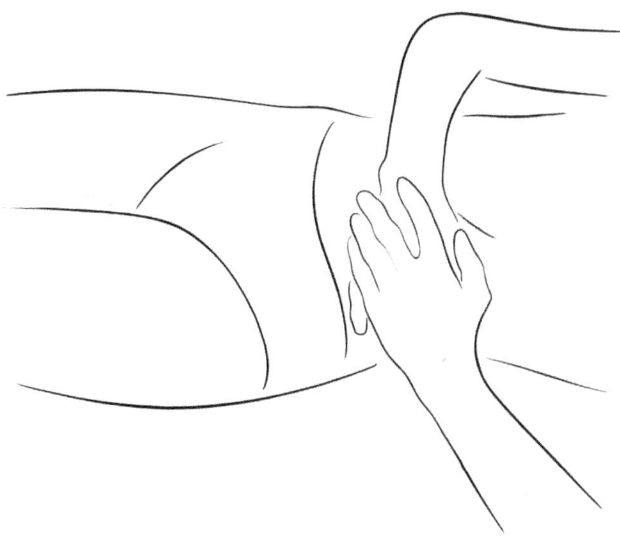

you regain your waistline faster after childbirth. You can start doing it from the first day. While lying on your back, slide one hand under your back on the opposite side. Slowly and gently glide your palm along the skin, stretching the muscles from your back to your belly button. Please perform this simple practice slowly and for a long duration, **without using oil**. Smooth out each side of your waist up to your belly button 40 times in a row.

After a cesarean section, skip this exercise.

- Pay special attention to your abdomen. To help your internal organs return to their place faster, I recommend performing a very simple self-massage called *Daisy* from the first day after vaginal childbirth.

In the case of a cesarean section, any massages and self-massages should only be started after the incision has healed (around one and a half to two months after giving birth) and after consulting with a doctor.

Daisy is a safe practice. It can become your daily ritual for many years ahead, as it improves women's health at any age. This self-massage is done for a considerable duration, ideally completing several rounds in one session.

Imagine that a daisy is drawn on your abdomen, with the navel as the center and the petals reaching the edges of your abdomen (under the ribs, down to the pubic area, and to the sides).

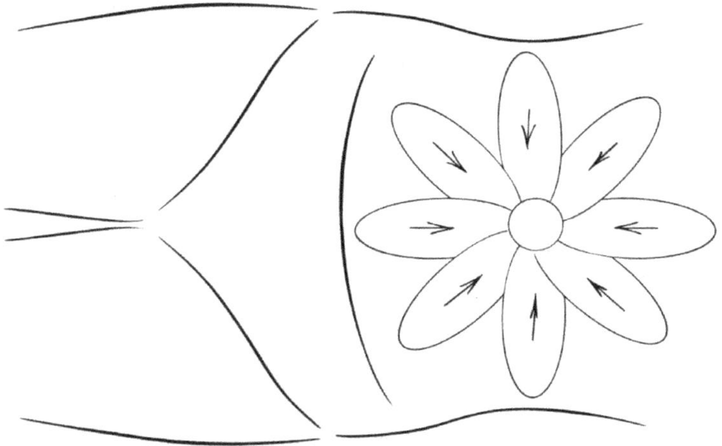

Place the palm of your right hand on the upper part of your abdomen, at the tip of the first 'petal'. Place your left hand on top. Wait for a moment to let the skin under your palm warm up. Then begin sliding from the tip of the 'petal' towards the center (the navel), keeping your hand attached to the skin as if it's glued to it.

Next, place your palms at the tip of the second petal (counterclockwise from the solar plexus) and slowly pull the 'glued' hand towards the navel. Then move on to the third petal and continue stroking your entire abdomen, petal by petal. The more petals your daisy has, the better. Pay special attention to the areas under the ribs (pancreas, liver).

Avoid touching the area of the uterus in the first few days, and especially after a cesarian – let the incision heal first. After a few days, you can gently stroke the petals and include the lower part of the abdomen.

Once again, I want to emphasize that after completing one round of massage, you can move on to the second, then the third — do as many rounds as you find enjoyable and comfortable. Give this exercise a try! You'll fall in love with it, just like I did. It has become my favorite body practice.

Practice breathing exercises

After vaginal childbirth, it's beneficial to engage in breathing exercises from the first day to initiate the body's recovery processes. Of course, do these exercises while lying on your back.

Place your palms on your lower ribs. Breathe using your chest, expanding your ribs on inhalation, and contracting on exhalation. Let your palms accompany this natural movement of the ribs during breathing. Do not exert any additional effort or force. Breathe through your nose, slowly and calmly. Five minutes of these breathing exercise will be sufficient!

After a cesarean section, breathing exercises are also very beneficial. In this case, lie on your back, place your hands on your lower ribs, and breathe using your abdomen. During inhalation, let your abdomen slightly inflate, and during exhalation, let it deflate. Use your hands to ensure that the ribs remain still during this process. Inhale and exhale through your nose, maintaining a calm breath.

Breathing exercises are generally beneficial for everyone regardless of age or life situation. However, after childbirth, I recommend practicing them for at least the first few days, especially when many of your muscles are still weak, and you spend most of your time in bed.

Apply castor oil compresses

This procedure, which comes from Balinese midwife Robin Lim, can be done from the first day after vaginal childbirth and two weeks after a cesarean section, without touching the suture area.

A castor oil compress helps reduce swelling, improve blood circulation, and has a lymphatic drainage effect. After several sessions, the skin of the abdomen becomes very soft and pleasant, and the abdomen itself returns to its pre-pregnancy size more quickly.

For postpartum recovery, it is recommended to do castor oil compresses two to three times a week for the first month. It is important to use specifically food-grade castor oil.

How to apply a compress. Ask someone close to you to warm up about 20ml of castor oil in a water bath (simply place the container with castor oil in a glass of hot water for a few minutes). At the same time, have a warm water bottle and a cotton cloth prepared for you.

Once the oil is warmed up, apply it to your abdomen and generously massage the abdominal skin with castor oil, including the area of the liver and pancreas. Cover your abdomen with the cotton cloth and place the warm water bottle on top. After 20-30 minutes (please, no longer! It's better to set a timer), remove the oil from your abdomen using the cloth. The procedure is finished. It's highly favorable to rest in bed or even go to sleep for some time now.

HOW TO START RESTORING BLOOD

Do you remember at the beginning of this section I told you about the three important tasks of the early postpartum period? You already know how to help the uterus contract and how to help the body heal. The third important task after childbirth is to start replenishing the blood.

Out of the five grams of iron we have before pregnancy, one gram is used for placenta formation, fetal growth, doubling the blood volume, and childbirth! During breastfeeding, an additional one microgram of iron is used daily for milk production. That's why there is a high risk of developing iron-deficiency anemia after childbirth. And that's why our priority is to start restoring blood through quality sleep and nutrition from the very first day.

Sleep is crucial for the prevention and treatment of anemia. During the first few days after childbirth, the mother should primarily eat, sleep, and rest with her baby in bed. Please pay special attention to sleep. The critical hours for sleep are from 11pm to 2am, as it is during this time that the liver synthesizes blood. Fortunately, even if the baby wakes up frequently at night, newborns usually sleep well during this period. If you are unable to get enough sleep at night, make sure to make up for the missing hours through daytime napping.

WHAT TO EAT FOR RECOVERY

Recovery nutrition after childbirth is a broad topic, but I'll give you the basics of postpartum nutrition. They are quite simple:

During the first forty days after childbirth, **the focus shifts from raw foods to cooked ones**. This is truly important. Your digestion is weakened after childbirth, and the better the food is cooked, the less energy your body will spend on digesting it. So, if you want to eat fruits or vegetables, try baking or steaming them.

Food after childbirth should be **warm**. Always remember how important warmth is for your recovery! The same applies to your food!

Food after childbirth should be **oily**. This will also improve your digestion and nourish you from the inside.

After childbirth, food should be **liquid and soft**. If you have grains, make them soupy. If you have vegetables, cook them well. Pureed soups, vegetable purees, baked fruits and vegetables, meatballs, and patties – these are ideal for postpartum nutrition.

Postpartum food should be **blood-nourishing**. We started this section by emphasizing the need to restore blood after childbirth. Well, you should do that primarily through the food you eat.

Foods to promote blood nourishment:
- Red meat
- Offal (especially liver)
- Long-cooked bone broths (recipe in the next chapter)
- Rooibos tea (3 cups a day contain the daily iron requirement)
- Natural pomegranate juice
- Blood-nourishing berries and their compotes (goji berries, red and black currants, raspberries, cherries, strawberries, gooseberries, jujube)
- Blood-nourishing fruits and dried fruits (plums, apples, pineapples, pears, apricots, figs).

Recipe for nettle infusion by Olga Kapustina

This drink is also very helpful in treating iron-deficiency anemia. However, it can only be prepared during the season: late spring to early summer.

Ingredients

Warm water – 3 liters
Nettle – 1 bunch
Strawberries – a few berries
Honey – a few tablespoons

Place all the ingredients in a jar, cover with gauze, and let it infuse for three days in a warm and sunny place. After three days, strain the infusion and store it in the refrigerator. Before consuming, the drink can be warmed slightly.

Knowing the main principles of postpartum nutrition, it will be easy for you to plan your own menu. Please do this in advance and ask your loved ones to take care of your food. Since you'll be lying down in the first few days after giving birth, someone else should take care of you and prepare restorative meals for you.

Please avoid going on any diets after childbirth, whether for weight loss or to prevent colic or allergies in your baby. A diet can undermine your health. After giving birth, you need a balanced diet that will meet your increased needs for vitamins and minerals. The only things you should truly exclude are listed below:

- Alcohol in any form and quantity
- White sugar
- Trans fats
- Products with chemicals (colorings, flavorings, preservatives, etc.)
- Products that you **personally** or your partner/baby's father are allergic to
- Products that **personally** cause bloating.

And the last thing I want to tell you in this chapter about food is the formula for postpartum nutrition, which goes like this:

> **Every meal = protein + fat + fiber**

1. You need to include protein in every meal. Hemoglobin, which binds iron, is a protein. If there's insufficient protein in the body, there won't be anything for iron to attach to.

   Where can you get protein from?
   - Animal protein
   - Fish
   - Seafood
   - Meat
   - Offal (liver, tongue, heart, sweetbreads)
   - Eggs

- Dairy products (except for sour cream and butter, as they are fats)

Plant protein:
- Legumes (but they need to be combined with rice or another grain to form a complete protein)
- Nuts (same as legumes)
- Nut milk (coconut, almond, pine nut, walnut)
- Buckwheat
- Quinoa
- Tofu
- Spirulina

If you're a vegetarian, focus on these protein sources.

2. You also need to include healthy fats in every meal. Your breast milk consists of 3-5% fat, so please consume something from this list daily:
   - Fatty fish
   - Lard (rendered fat)
   - Nuts (preferably soaked)
   - Seeds (sesame and flax seeds need to be ground before consumption for better absorption)
   - Olives
   - Olive oil
   - Coconut oil
   - Flaxseed oil
   - Pumpkin seed oil
   - Avocado
   - Ghee (clarified butter)
   - Sour cream

3. You need fiber in every meal for healthy digestion. Please make sure to include whole grains (such as whole grain rice, whole oats, barley, buckwheat, quinoa, and products made from whole grain flour), fruits, and vegetables in your daily diet – but make sure they are cooked thoroughly.

You also need **energy for digestion and recovery**! Energy-rich foods include well-cooked, easily digestible porridges (the best options for this purpose are corn, barley, oat, and wheat porridges), which should be consumed daily after childbirth. In addition, bone broths provide energy (please drink at least one cup per week, but you can have a cup every day), as well as long-cooked fruit compotes. You will find the recipes for these in the next chapter.

Here's a recipe for a **restorative soup** by Anhelina Martinez, which is ideal as the first meal you can have right after childbirth.

If you're a vegetarian, focus on green vegetables – a variety of greens that are rich in iron – rather than chicken. Don't forget about spices, as they are also relevant for you!

> *If you had a cesarean section, the principles of postpartum nutrition described above are equally important for you. Pay even more attention to foods that help with blood formation because you will have lost more blood during the operation. Additionally, for faster and better wound healing,*

it's important to consume foods rich in collagen, such as fish and meat bone broths (recipe in the next chapter), aspic, eggs, gelatin, and seafood. To enhance the absorption of collagen (and iron), incorporate foods high in vitamin C into your diet, such as citrus fruits, strawberries, spinach, sweet peppers, rosehips, and tart berries.

Restorative soup

Ingredients

Water
Organic chicken (if you are a vegetarian, there will be an alternative below) Spices: garlic, onion, basil, rosemary, thyme, and oregano
Oil (ghee is the best option)
Potatoes
Carrots
Various green vegetables (zucchini, bell pepper, broccoli, beet greens)

First, prepare the chicken broth (see the recipe in the chapter *Restorative beverage recipes*). If the chicken is not organic, discard the first water after 20 minutes of boiling. Then, sauté the spices in oil. Add potatoes, carrots, and all the available green vegetables to the broth, depending on the season. Cook the vegetables until tender. When the soup has cooled, blend it using a blender.

Please note that it's essential to consult with your healthcare provider or a nutritionist for personalized advice based on your specific dietary needs and medical history.

RESTORATIVE BEVERAGE RECIPES

I have mentioned many times the importance of consuming restorative beverages after childbirth. It would be wonderful if you could have **infusions of blood-boosting berries or dried fruits**, and **rooibos tea** prepared for you every day, and once a week a long-cooked **bone broth** rich in amino acids and collagen. These three types of beverages are the foundation for postpartum recovery.

It's great if you add spices to your postpartum beverages (any kind). The best **spices for the postpartum period** are turmeric and cinnamon (these are basic spices that will be suitable even if you are not familiar with spices), fenugreek, rosemary, fennel, anise, ginger, cumin, saffron, cardamom, cloves, black pepper, and red pepper. All of them are suitable for breastfeeding. Spices after childbirth help to address many issues.

Improve digestion
- Turmeric
- Cumin

- Ginger
- Anise
- Fennel

Strengthen uterine contractions

- Cinnamon
- Saffron
- Rosemary

Increase lactation

- Fennel
- Cumin
- Fenugreek
- Cinnamon

Provide warmth

- Turmeric
- Ginger
- Rosemary
- Fenugreek
- Red pepper

Benefit the nervous system

- Saffron
- Cardamom
- Cloves (has a sedative effect)

Have antiseptic and antibacterial properties

- Turmeric
- Cloves
- Fenugreek

Attention: Always use spices in very small quantities, as instructed! Consuming large amounts of spices at once can have negative side effects! It is also important to use spices separately: one spice for one beverage (unless otherwise specified in the recipe), at least in the beginning. If a spice is new to you, introduce it into your diet carefully and observe your body's reaction for several days.

Recipe for berry/dried fruit infusion by Alena Lebedeva

Ingredients:

Water – 1 liter

Berries/fruits/dried fruits (goji berries, viburnum, red and black currants, raspberries, cherries, strawberries, gooseberries, jujube, plum, apple, pineapple, pear, apricot, fig)

A pinch of spice (choose from the above list)

For 1 liter of water, take a handful (or two to three, for a more concentrated infusion) of any berries or dried fruits. The more ingredients you have in the beverage, the better.

Bring the water to a boil, add the berries, fruits, and/or dried fruits, and simmer over low heat for 20-30 minutes. Then add the spice and simmer for another 5-10 minutes. Pour into a thermos to keep the beverage hot.

Express version

If you don't have the opportunity to prepare a decoction, you can do it this way: put a handful of berries in a thermos, pour boiling water over them, and let them steep overnight. You can drink it in the morning.

Recipe for bone broth

Ingredients:

Water – 3 liters
Bones (chicken/beef/lamb/fish), preferably from organic animals – 0.8-1kg
Natural apple cider vinegar – 1 tbsp
Carrot – 1
Onion – 1
Celery stalk – 1
Garlic – 3 cloves
Bay leaf – 2 leaves
Black peppercorns – a few
Salt – 1 tsp

Bone broth is prepared from bones. If you don't have bones, you can take meat on the bone, boil it, and then remove it from the bone. Use the bones themselves to cook the healing broth.

Ideally, the bones should be from organic (home-raised) animals. If unsure about the origin of the meat, boil for 20 minutes first then pour out the water.

Cover the prepared bones with fresh water, add apple cider vinegar, raw vegetables, and spices.

Place the pot on the stove, bring it to a boil, then reduce the heat to a level where the broth barely simmers. Cook for 6-12 hours. When the broth is ready, strain it from the vegetables and spices, let it cool, and store it in the refrigerator for up to five days.

You can drink the broth as is, one cup per day, or add it to any food. Excess broth can be frozen.

Recipe for plant-based milk

I didn't include plant-based milk in the top three basic postpartum beverages, but it is very beneficial as it contains protein and many vitamins. Plant-based milk can be made from coconut flakes, almonds, walnuts, pine nuts, sesame seeds, or sunflower seeds.

Ingredients:

Water – 3 cups
Nuts or seeds – 1 cup

Soak a cup of nuts or seeds in water overnight. In the morning, drain the water and place the soaked nuts or seeds in a blender (if making almond milk, remove the skins from the almonds). Add water in a ratio of 1(nuts/seeds):3(Water). Blend everything for a few minutes, then strain the mixture through a sieve or cheesecloth to remove the pulp, and drink the milk.

Express version

Plant-based milk can be made even easier and faster using nut butter. Mix 2-3 tablespoons of nut butter with a cup of water in a blender. The milk is ready.

You can use plant-based milk to cook porridge, soups, drink it as is, or make a chocolate beverage by adding carob.

Recipe for chocolate beverage

Ingredients:
Plant-based milk – 1 cup
Carob syrup – 1 tbsp

Heat the plant-based milk and add the carob syrup. Stir until the syrup is completely dissolved.

Carob syrup helps restore blood composition, boosts immunity, improves digestion, has a positive effect on the nervous system, promotes better sleep, and strengthens bone tissues. It is effective in treating anemia after childbirth (as part of comprehensive therapy).

Carob syrup is extracted from carob pods without using sugar! It is truly a unique product that is recommended even for pregnant women and children from the age of two. You can dilute carob syrup in water, but it is tastier and more nutritious in plant-based milk. I would be delighted if you discover this beneficial treat.

Recipe for cocoa beverage by Anhelina Martinez

In Mexico, cocoa beans are considered one of the main foods for pregnancy, childbirth, and recovery. Traditional Mexican midwives give women a cup of homemade chocolate or another beverage made from cocoa beans to drink immediately after childbirth. Make sure this recipe for cocoa beans is in your collection!

Ingredients:

Water – 3 liters

Cocoa beans – 100g (if you don't have beans, you can use 100g cocoa powder + 1tbsp of ghee)

Oatmeal – to taste and preference (optional)

Honey

First, roast the cocoa beans for about 5 minutes. Then peel them and soak them in water for 3 hours. After that, blend everything in a blender, and optionally add oatmeal as a thickener. Bring the mixture to a boil and simmer for 3-4 minutes. When the beverage cools down, add a little honey.

Recipe for orange drink by Olga Kapustina

Ingredients:
    Water – 2 cups
    Orange – 1
    Turmeric, rosemary or other spice

Boil the water and let it cool slightly. Add the juice form the orange and your spice of choice. The drink is ready.

This drink, like the previous one made from cocoa beans, improves mood and serves as a preventive measure against postpartum depression. If you and your baby's father do not have allergies to oranges or cocoa, you can safely consume both drinks while breastfeeding.

May these postpartum drinks make your recovery not only quick but also delicious!

PSYCHOLOGICAL RECOVERY AFTER A DIFFICULT CHILDBIRTH

My dear, if your childbirth did not go according to plan, I'm so sorry... I empathize with you deeply... I know how challenging it can be to accept, how much strength and time it can take to process this loss: the loss of your expectations for childbirth, the loss of your vision of a perfect birth.

You **have the right to all your feelings**. Please, experience them. And if you feel like crying, please, **go ahead and cry**. Tears release. If you feel that it's difficult for you to cope with this, please seek help from a perinatal psychologist. It's normal. It's not shameful. It's safe. It works.

If you feel like talking about your childbirth with someone, please do so: ask your husband, mother, or friend (someone who loves you and whom you trust) to listen to you silently, without comments or advice, and **tell this person about your childbirth**. Repeat the same story over and over until you feel it becomes easier.

If you have any unanswered questions after childbirth, please try **reframing these questions**. Take your time and reflect on each new phrase...

Why couldn't my body handle it?

My body did handle it! It conceived, carried, and *gave birth* to a child! What can I do for it as a gesture of love and gratitude?

Why couldn't I handle it?

I did handle it! I *did everything I could* and more, and my experience is even more valuable because I had to endure a lot of pain. What good things can I do for myself? What gift can I give myself to mark my greatest success? I have given new life!

Why did everything happen this way?

What good came out of my childbirth?
What could I have done differently?
What have I learned from my childbirth?

Why did this happen to me?

Could I have learned all the things I learned in childbirth as quickly and effectively through some other means?

And there's something else I want to ask of you. Please, **look forward, not backward**. Later, when you have more strength and at a more suitable time, you will definitely come to terms with everything that happened during your childbirth. But right now... you have your baby, a wonderful, and hopefully healthy child. Your baby needs you. They need you completely. They need you to make them the sole focus of all your thoughts and feelings.

Let the childbirth wait a bit. You will definitely come back to it. Focus on what is happening in your life **right now**, on your baby and their needs. After all, in the end, pregnancy and childbirth happen so that a new person, your child, is born. And if everything is going well with them, let that be your **greatest success** right now. A greater success than the process of childbirth itself. Because you didn't go through labor just for the process, but for this wonderful result that is hopefully lying next to you, sleeping soundly.

I embrace you, my dear. How I wish I could hug you right now!

BREASTFEEDING

My dear, I truly hope that you will breastfeed your baby (or at least give it a try). It won't make your breasts worse or less attractive. On the contrary, breastfeeding is very beneficial for you – it's a powerful prevention against breast and ovarian cancer. And for your little one, your breast milk is the best, most nutritious, and most delicious food they can have. No formula can compete with your milk because formula contains only a small percentage of breast milk's components.

If you understand the significance of these facts and want to try breastfeeding your child, know that you have a 95% chance of being able to do so based on your physiology. The idea of 'milk' and 'non-milk' women is nothing more than a myth. A healthy mother who has breasts can inherently nourish her baby! It only requires basic knowledge, willingness, and some effort.

I must warn you that breastfeeding is an art, as well as a whole science that you will learn day by day. It may take time for both you and your baby to get the hang of it, and you may encounter challenges along the way. But with support and perseverance, you can establish a beautiful and nourishing breastfeeding relationship with your little one.

Remember, breastfeeding is not just about nutrition, it's also about bonding, comfort, and emotional connection between you and your baby. Take it one step at a time, seek guidance if needed, and trust your instincts. You are capable of providing the best for your baby, and your breastfeeding journey can be a beautiful and fulfilling experience.

Perhaps you will encounter difficulties, but believe me, any challenges can be overcome. Nowadays, there are breastfeeding consultants available in almost every city. You can confidently trust them. Be sure to reach out to a consultant if you're having trouble establishing lactation. The earlier you do it, the easier it will be to correct any mistakes. Time is working against you in this matter.

Since my book is dedicated to childbirth and the early days after birth, I will only tell you about lactation as it relates to this time. Specifically, how to establish breastfeeding, how to help your milk come in faster, what to do in case of engorgement, and how to treat nipple cracks.

HOW TO ESTABLISH LACTATION

It is crucial to put your baby to the breast within the first hour after birth to establish lactation. Your baby may not immediately want to latch or may latch but not feed. Keep trying (without force) to offer the breast again and again until they want to suckle.

The success of your breastfeeding will depend, to a large extent, on **how correctly you position your baby at the**

breast. This will affect the amount of milk you have, the presence of nipple cracks, whether your baby is getting enough nourishment, and their weight gain.

How to properly position your baby at the breast

Support your breast with your hand like a cup when offering it to your baby.

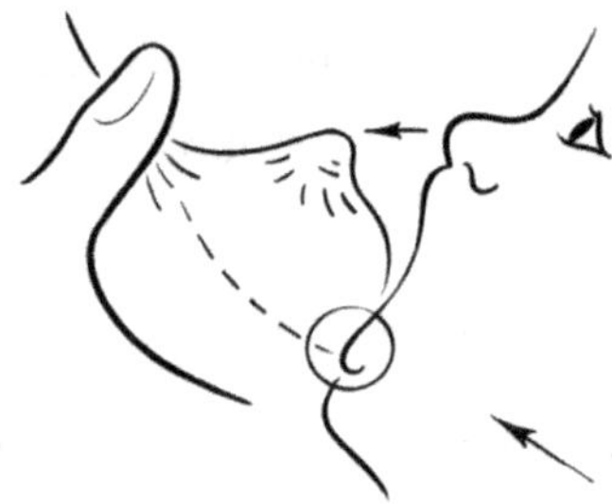

Aim the nipple toward your baby's nose.

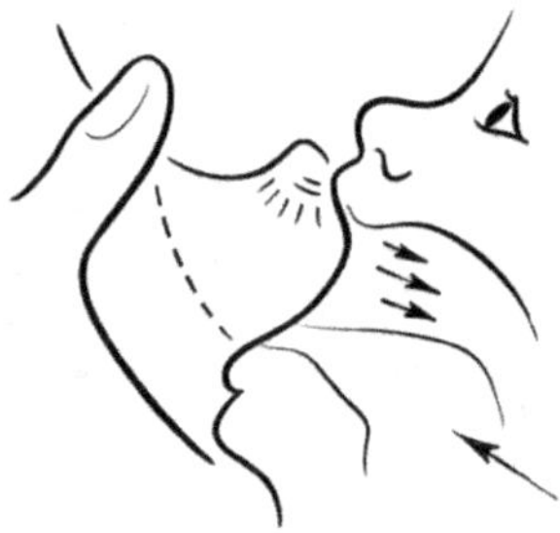

Your nipple should be slightly pointing upward. Before your baby latches, you can gently pull back on the breast skin with your thumb to encourage a good latch.

To offer your breast, place the nipple against your baby's upper lip. They will tilt their head back and latch onto the nipple correctly.

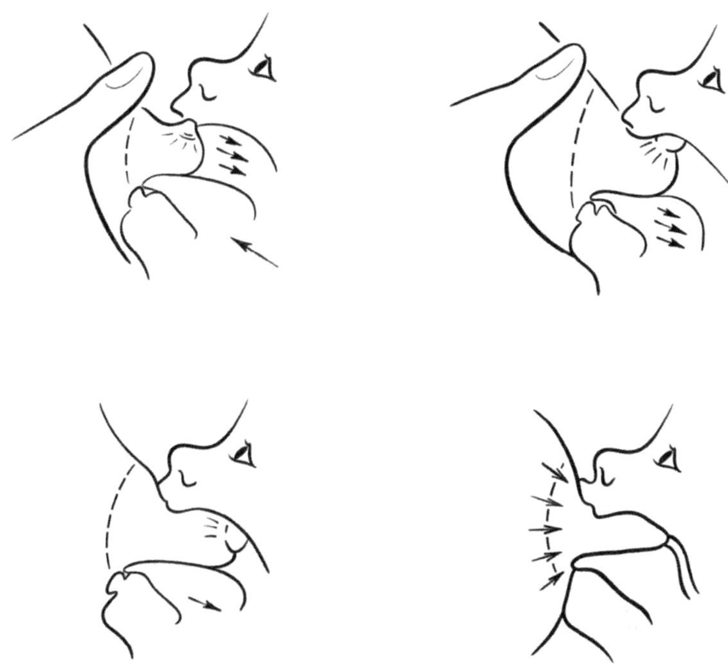

How to know if you have latched correctly

- Your baby's belly is pressed against you, even if you are breastfeeding while lying down.

- Your baby's chin is pressed against your breast.

- Their mouth is wide open, with the lower lip turned outward.

- You can see a little bit of your areola above the baby's mouth, while the bottom part is fully inside their mouth.

- There are no extra sounds during feeding, such as smacking or sucking in air.

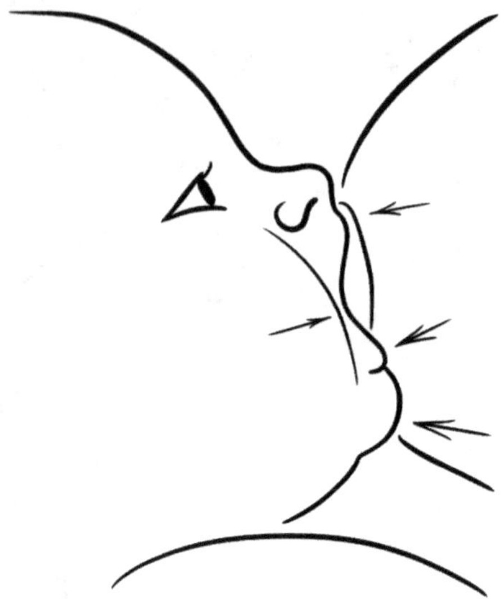

Best positions for initial latch

1. Lying on your side

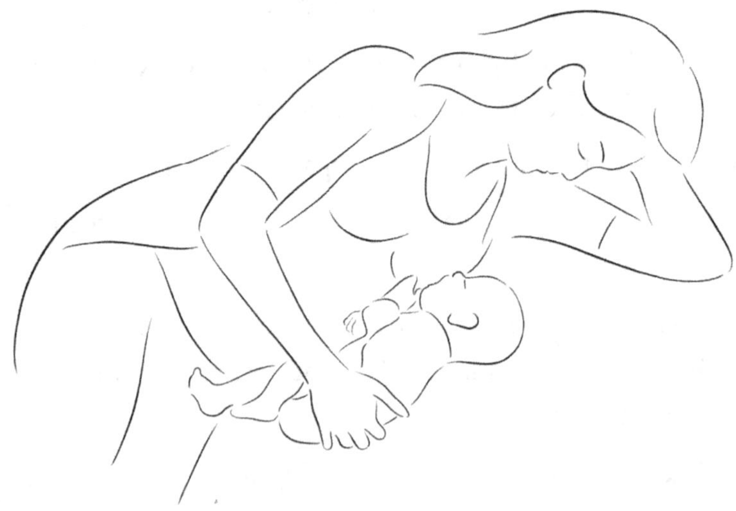

2. Sitting or semi-sitting (cradle hold and cross-cradle hold)

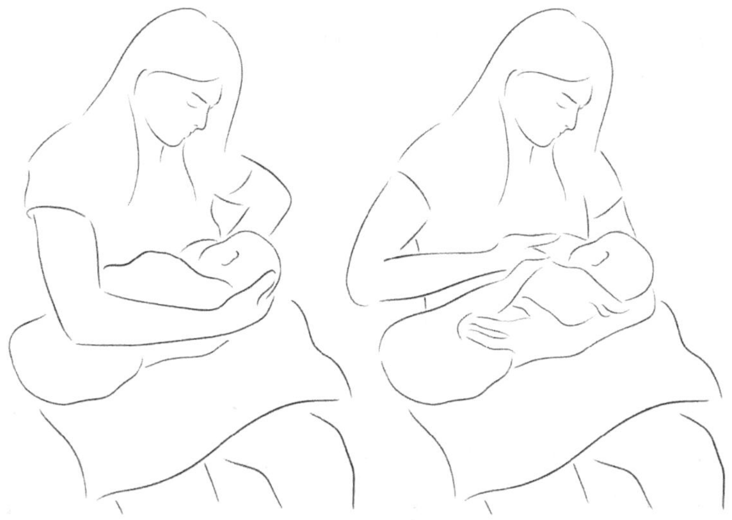

3. Sitting or semi-sitting underarm hold.

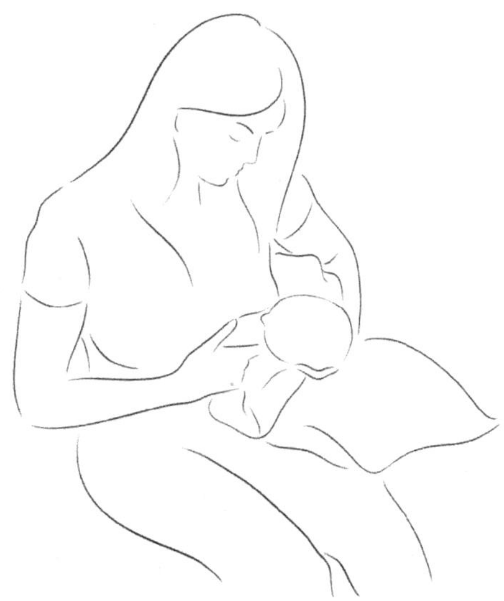

In general, there are many more positions for breastfeeding. Once you have mastered these basic positions and established lactation, you can try any other positions that are comfortable for you.

Other important guidelines for establishing lactation

1. Feed your baby on demand (when they open their mouth, search for the breast, grunt, or cry), rather than following a strict schedule. Feeding on a schedule is an outdated recommendation that many doctors no longer support. Trust your baby's cues to determine when to offer the breast. Even if only 10 minutes have passed since the last feeding and they are asking for the breast again, it is normal. Once lactation is established, you will develop a feeding routine, and the intervals between feedings will become longer.

2. Avoid long gaps between feedings. In the first month after childbirth, the maximum gap between feedings should be two hours. If your baby sleeps for more than two hours in that first month, wake them up and offer the breast. If there is a long gap between feedings (four hours or more), the newborn's blood sugar level can drop so much that they might not have the energy to wake up and ask for food.

3. Do not restrict the time your baby spends at the breast. Some babies eat quickly, while others enjoy sucking for longer periods. Don't worry about it. Focus on your own baby. Even if your baby falls asleep at the breast,

they may still be nursing during that time. If you are sure they have finished feeding, gently insert your pinky finger between your breast and the baby's mouth. This will release the vacuum created during feeding, allowing the baby to easily release the nipple without causing any harm.

4. Change breasts for each feeding, but not more frequently than every one and a half to two hours. If you have fed your baby and they ask for the breast again shortly after, offer the same breast. To remember which breast you last fed from, attach a safety pin to your clothing on the side you nursed from, and after feeding from the other breast, move the safety pin to the opposite side.

5. Avoid using pacifiers and bottles in the first month after childbirth. They are the main enemies of breastfeeding and can disrupt the establishment of lactation. You can start using them after forty days postpartum. If there is a need to supplement your baby's feeding with expressed milk or formula in the first month, use a syringe without needle or spoon for that purpose.

6. Do not use formula in the first few days after childbirth. Until your milk comes in, your baby will have enough colostrum. They are not starving, and they will not die of hunger. Yes, they may lose some weight, but losing up to 10% of their birth weight is normal and does not require supplementation with formula. If the baby cries in the first few days after birth, it is not always because

they are hungry (nature has provided newborns with subcutaneous fat reserves, and in the first few days, they do not need more than a few drops of colostrum). Newborn crying can have many different reasons, not just hunger.

7. Relax and wait for your milk to come in. Don't panic! Normally, milk comes in within the first seven days (!) after childbirth, but more commonly on the third day. To help your milk come in faster, breastfeed your baby more frequently, eat well, drink plenty of warm fluids (water, teas, and other postpartum drinks), and follow all the recommendations mentioned above.

8. Create conditions for milk production. The main hormones for lactation are prolactin and oxytocin. For the first, it's important to have mechanical stimulation of the nipple and areola receptors, quality sleep, and rest. For the second, create a warm, dark, and quiet environment that promotes a sense of safety, stimulate the nipples, have privacy with your baby, and allow yourself to enjoy your motherhood and breastfeeding experience.

9. Do not pump your breasts if your baby doesn't have any issues with latching. Pumping after each feed, often called 'emptying the breast', is as outdated a recommendation as feeding on schedule. It can lead to oversupply (producing too much milk), which can be difficult to manage, and potentially cause breast trauma if done incorrectly. Moreover, it is a time-consuming and often unnecessary activity.

WHAT TO DO IF YOU HAVE LOW MILK SUPPLY

Your body is intelligent! It knows how much milk your baby needs. If you follow all the rules for establishing breastfeeding, your body should produce enough milk to satisfy your baby's needs.

If, despite your efforts to breastfeed on demand and latch correctly, you still have low milk supply, the following tips may help:

- Get more sleep and rest.
- Find ways to relax (take a bath, have someone give you a massage).
- Consume foods and beverages that promote blood production (milk is produced from your blood).
- Drink hot beverages (it can stimulate lactation).
- Eat buckwheat and carrots (known as lactogenic foods).
- Try black cumin oil (1 teaspoon of oil mixed with 1 teaspoon of honey, taken once a day after meals, for no more than a month).
- Add herbs and spices for lactation to your diet (fenugreek, nettle, fennel, dill seed, cumin, cinnamon).

Keep in mind that mint and sage significantly decrease lactation, so avoid them while breastfeeding your baby.

NIPPLE CRACKS

The most common cause of nipple trauma is an incorrect latch. Therefore, for prevention and when cracks already appear, it's essential to improve the latch. If you're unable to do it yourself, please consider seeking help from a lactation consultant. They can also check if your baby has a short frenulum, as that can contribute to the formation of cracks.

The best remedy for nipple cracks is airing nipples out and applying your own breast milk to them after each feeding. In addition to breast milk, you can also apply either lanolin, Solcoseryl, narrow-leaved lavender essential oil (either undiluted or diluted in a carrier oil), or diluted geranium essential oil (one drop of essential oil per one teaspoon of carrier oil) after each feeding.

Until the cracks heal, minimize (or better yet, completely avoid) contact between your nipples and water. Water can dry out the skin and slow down the healing process.

LACTOSTASIS

Often, when milk first comes in, breastfeeding mothers face the problem of breast engorgement. The breasts become full and firm, causing discomfort. When the baby feeds and consumes some milk, the pressure is relieved, and the breast becomes softer and lighter as it empties evenly.

But sometimes, even after a feeding, when the baby has consumed milk, a small or large area of the breast remains firm. This firmness does not go away after one or two feedings and can persist for several days. This condition is called a lactostasis or milk stasis. Don't worry, every breastfeeding mother sooner or later encounters this, and sometimes more than once.

The alveoli, which produce milk, are connected to ducts in the breast, forming a common milk duct. With lactostasis, one of these ducts may become blocked, preventing the release of milk and causing it to build up. Milk continues to be produced and enters the breast, but a milk plug, formed by a clump of fat, prevents the milk from easily exiting. It moves very slowly during breastfeeding.

Why does this fat clot suddenly block the duct? During the pause between feedings, fat particles from the milk adhere to the walls of the ducts. When the baby breastfeeds, a fresh influx of milk pushes this fat toward the exit. However, if the duct has narrowed for some reason, the fat particles can block the passage. There can be several reasons for this phenomenon: an excess of milk, maternal stress (adrenaline release into the bloodstream), excessive physical exertion or lifting heavy objects, wearing uncomfortable or tight bras, and overall tight clothing.

In the first few days after childbirth, lactostasis can also occur after rough pumping. Forceful or rough expression can damage the breast tissue, leading to swelling. This swelling increases and becomes painful, and the skin on the breast may even turn red.

What to do if you experience lactostasis

1. *Before* each feeding, if you don't have a fever, apply a warm compress to the area of hardness on your breast (a water bottle, a bag of warm grains, a warmed blanket). Heat expands the ducts, making it easier for milk to flow.

2. Immediately after that, latch your baby to the breast, feed, and then remove the baby.

3. *After* each feeding, apply cold to the breast. This reduces milk production in the future. You can use a frozen pack or an ice cube from the freezer and hold it on your breast for five minutes. You will quickly feel relief! Some doctors advise against applying cold to the breast, fearing that it may cause a cold. In reality, that's not the case. When we have a bruise or injury to any part of the body, we apply ice without catching a cold. It's a different matter that women with lactostasis may have a weakened immune system and may be more prone to catching a cold, but ice is not the cause!

4. After the cold treatment, apply a refrigerated cabbage leaf to the problem area and keep it there until it

becomes wilted, then replace it with a fresh one. You can continue this process until the hardness resolves.

What else can help?

- Position your baby at the breast so that their chin touches the area of hardness. This way, while nursing, the baby will massage the hardness. (You can find many different breastfeeding positions online.)
- Breastfeed your baby as frequently as possible. If you can't latch the baby, express a little milk using gentle, soft motions. Apply gentle pressure to the areola and lightly massage around the nipple. Avoid pressing down on the breast from the top. Express milk only until you feel the tension release. This is important! Otherwise, the breast will continue producing more milk, repeatedly.
- If the hardness is only in one breast, give that breast more attention. Instead of alternating breasts after each feeding, feed the affected breast three or four times in a row, then feed the healthy breast once, and repeat the cycle.
- As soon as you feel the milk let-down, immediately latch your baby to the breast, even if they are asleep (wake them up). If you cannot latch the baby, express milk until the tension is relieved. Sometimes there can be an excess of milk, and the baby may not be able to consume it all during feeding. In that case,

express a little milk before feeding so that the baby can primarily suck on the hardness.

I also recommend calling a lactation consultant to come to your home for breastfeeding support if you're experiencing lactostasis.

What to do if you develop a fever during lactostasis

First of all, continue breastfeeding your baby! No one except your baby can effectively empty your breast, and frequent emptying is crucial during lactostasis. You can continue breastfeeding even if you have a fever. If you're feeling fine, there's no need to lower your temperature.

An elevated body temperature during lactostasis may be accompanied by redness on the skin of the breast, which suggests that the swelling may progress to mastitis and become infected. Therefore, if you have a fever, avoid applying any heat to your breast. Avoid using alcohol compresses, physical therapies (as they can stimulate milk flow), or Vishnevsky ointment.

If lactostasis occurs with a fever, the key is frequent feedings and applying ice to the breast for five minutes after each feeding. If you are expressing milk, apply gentle pressure to the breast and avoid pressing on the areas with lumps. Try to empty your breast as often as possible.

Can you use a breast pump during lactostasis?

Only very expensive breast pumps work in a way similar to a baby's suckling. Regular vacuum-based breast pumps may further damage the breast. Additionally, they increase the risk of infection. Therefore, it's better to hand express milk. It is safer, more effective, and free!

Do you need to take antibiotics for lactostasis?

Not always, but you should consult with a doctor. Know that even if you need to take antibiotics, you can continue breastfeeding your baby.

Can lactostasis be prevented?

Certainly! To prevent the occurrence of lactostasis, you should:

- Wear loose-fitting clothing throughout the lactation period. Avoid tight bras, including nursing bras. If you wear a bra, choose one without underwire and always remove it before breastfeeding.

- Avoid using breast pads that hinder air circulation, as they increase the risk of nipple cracks and infection.

- Never fully empty the breast while expressing milk – only express until you feel the release of tension.

- Rest as much as possible, as it is essential for your health!

I believe that you can handle any challenges that may arise during lactation. And I sincerely hope that this book will help you avoid many issues. Wishing you success on this beautiful, incredible, and unparalleled journey of breastfeeding!

YOUR BABY

This book would be incomplete if I didn't dedicate at least a few lines to your little one. This is not just a small person – it's an entire universe that you now need to discover and understand!

After giving birth, you will have to learn everything externally: how to carry your baby, care for them, feed, bathe, put them to sleep, take them for walks, communicate with them, play, maintain their health, and provide treatment when needed. There are many books written on these topics, and I highly recommend that you read them.

However, I want to tell you that **one of the most important things you need to learn after giving birth is to understand your baby and respond to their needs**. This is the key to their emotional well-being. It may be the most challenging aspect for you in the beginning because your baby cannot speak, and crying is their only way of expressing that something is wrong.

And there can be many reasons for their crying. What is your little one trying to communicate through their cries?

- I'm hungry.
- I'm tired.
- I want to be held.
- Something is uncomfortable or itchy (they might be experiencing some discomfort).
- I need to pee/poop (or they have already done so).
- I feel like I've been forgotten.
- I'm anxious.
- I just want to cry (this can also happen, and it's normal).

How to understand why the little one is crying right now

Surprisingly, newborns cry for various reasons! This is where your task as a mother lies – to learn to understand what the baby wants to tell you through their cries.

Even if this is your first child, by carefully observing them during the first forty days after childbirth and studying their behavior, by around one and a half months old, you will learn to distinguish between a hungry cry and a sleepy one, a frightened cry and a painful one. Just listen to your intuition and be attuned to the baby's 'wave', then their language of communication will become accessible to you.

Do you know what a newborn baby needs from parents, especially from you?

- To be loved
- To be given a sense of security

- To have their needs met promptly and correctly (in the way they expect from you).

The main task during the first one and a half months of a baby's life is to understand what is happening with them and to do what they need. This is called parental competence. Understanding your little one is not enough. You also need to properly fulfill their needs. If the baby is hungry, they need to be breastfed. If their tummy hurts, they need to be comforted, helped to endure the pain, and relieved. In such cases, breastfeeding may not work and may even upset the baby because it is not what they are asking for or what they need right now.

No matter how significant breastfeeding is for an infant, you need to learn to solve 'issues' unrelated to food in other ways as well:
- Carry them in your arms
- Change their diaper
- Stroke them gently
- Speak to them softly
- Simply hug and comfort them
- Rock them, lull them to sleep, or help them fall asleep.

I know that parenting for the first time is not easy. But you have support: your family, friends, doctors, and professionals in helping fields (lactation consultants, sleep consultants, perinatal psychologists, postpartum doulas, osteopaths).

Dear one, be happy in your motherhood! I wholeheartedly wish you lots of love, joy, inspiration, and harmony on this journey. I'm not saying goodbye to you but rather, 'see you' on the pages of my other books, which I hope will be as useful to you as this one.

CONCLUSION

Dear mom, I have shared a lot with you on the pages of this book. Before we part ways, there's something else I want to tell you. Something important. This is my final message to you. If I could have spoken to myself when I was pregnant, I would have said the same words...

Dear one, you may consider childbirth as your exam, but how it unfolds depends not only on you but also on the destiny of your baby.

Dear one, if childbirth doesn't go as you desire, it doesn't mean you're a bad mother. It means your child had a different path.

Dear one, childbirth is just one day that quickly passes. Ahead lies a whole lifetime, and it's important to prepare for what awaits you and to avoid making mistakes.

Dear one, if something doesn't go as planned during childbirth, if there are interventions and difficulties, many things can be compensated for after birth. It's not the end of the world.

Dear one, take care of yourself after giving birth. Don't hesitate to ask for help, seek advice, and prioritize self-care. It's the foundation of a happy motherhood.

Dear one, you're a good mother no matter what, simply because you love your child and do everything you can for them.

 Ecaterina Mikitenko

Dear one, don't bear all the responsibility for your little one alone. Share it with their father, and grandparents, because they are just as much a part of the baby's life as you are.

Dear one, don't compare yourself to others or try to measure up. You have your own unique path in motherhood, and it's good enough for you and your child.

Dear one, you're not alone. There are dozens, hundreds, thousands of women who have been or are in similar situations. They've overcome, and so will you. I believe in you.

With much love for you and your little one,
Your doula, Ecaterina Mikitenko

GRATITUDE

With all my heart, I express my gratitude for the knowledge of all the specialists (doctors, midwives, doulas, psychotherapists) from whom I have learned so much:

Gertruda Shpatakovska for profound knowledge of perinatal psychology;

Alena Lebedeva for invaluable knowledge of the physiology of the postpartum period;

Michel Odent for fundamental knowledge about the physiology of childbirth and the basic needs of laboring women;

Daria Streltsova for practical knowledge of doula support during childbirth;

Stephanie Larson and **Ekaterina Grankina** for the amazing Dancing For Birth™ childbirth preparation program, some movements and principles of which I shared in the book;

Anghelina Martinez Miranda for wonderful birthing techniques and recipes for the postpartum period;

Svetlana Akimova for wise knowledge of gentle birth and gentle care for women;

Natalya Savelieva for knowledge in the field of aromatherapy and assistance in writing the chapter on essential oils for childbirth;

     Ecaterina Mikitenko

Julia Sliusareva for effective techniques for correcting cervical position during labor;

Olga Kapustina for useful recipes of postpartum restorative drinks and knowledge about the peculiarities of recovery after a cesarean section;

and **all the other teachers** I have encountered on my professional path who have helped birth this book in one way or another.

I am grateful to **all the women** who have approached me for their experiences.

I thank **my family** for their support.

I thank my husband, **Dmitrii Mikitenko**, for believing in me, assisting at every stage of creating the book, and especially for the illustrations and cover.

I thank **God** for life and inspiration.

May this book bring benefit to many women!

ABOUT THE AUTHOR

Ecaterina Mikitenko is a mother of two children, a certified perinatal fitness instructor for Dancing For Birth™, a prenatal and childbirth preparation course organizer, a doula, a certified intimate gymnastics coach, a symptothermal fertility awareness and natural family planning consultant, and an author of parenting books.

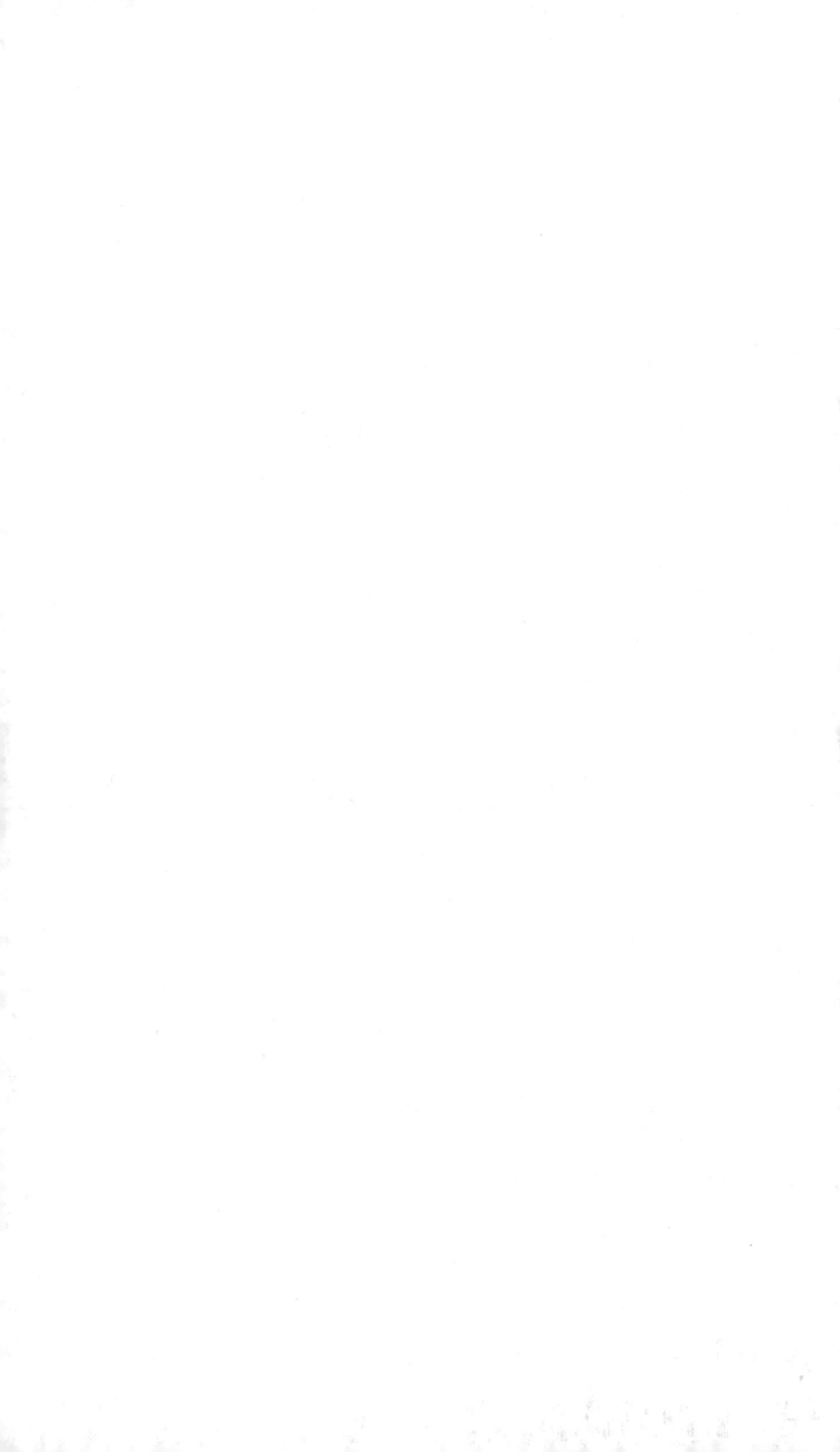